THE SMALL THINGS

THE SMALL THINGS

JAYNE HUGHES

Writing Dr

THE SMALL THINGS
By
JAYNE HUGHES BEM

First published in Great Britain by Writing Dr

www.writingdr.com

Copyright © 2025 Jayne Hughes BEM

All rights reserved.
No part of this publication may be reproduced, stored in a retrieval system, or transmitted in any form or by any means without the prior written permission of the publisher, nor be otherwise circulated in any form of binding or cover other than that in which it is published without a similar condition being imposed on the subsequent purchaser.

This book is for information or education purposes only. It is not a substitute for professional medical advice or treatment. Any person requiring medical attention should consult with a qualified healthcare professional. Always seek the advice of your physician or other qualified health provider with any questions you may have regarding a medical condition. Never disregard professional medical advice or delay in seeking it because of something you have read in this book.

Neither the author, contributors, nor the publisher shall be liable or responsible for any adverse effects or consequences allegedly arising directly or indirectly from the use of any information contained in this book. In the interest of confidentiality, some names and details have been changed. The opinions expressed in this book represent the personal views of the author and not of the publisher.

For every child whose bright light was dimmed too soon by a rare disease – your courage, laughter, and love leave footprints on our hearts.
For every parent and sibling who faces deep loss with such dignity, we salute you.
For every clinician and scientist who listens, dedicates their lives to others, we are grateful for you.

This book is especially dedicated to Amy, whose spirit continues to shine in every star, every story and every second – you taught us the meaning of strength, true love and life, and showed us the beauty of small joys daily.
You are forever missed, forever remembered, and forever loved.
Over and out sweet girlie…

"Enjoy the little things in life, for one day you may look back and realise they were the big things" Robert Brault and Kurt Vonnegut

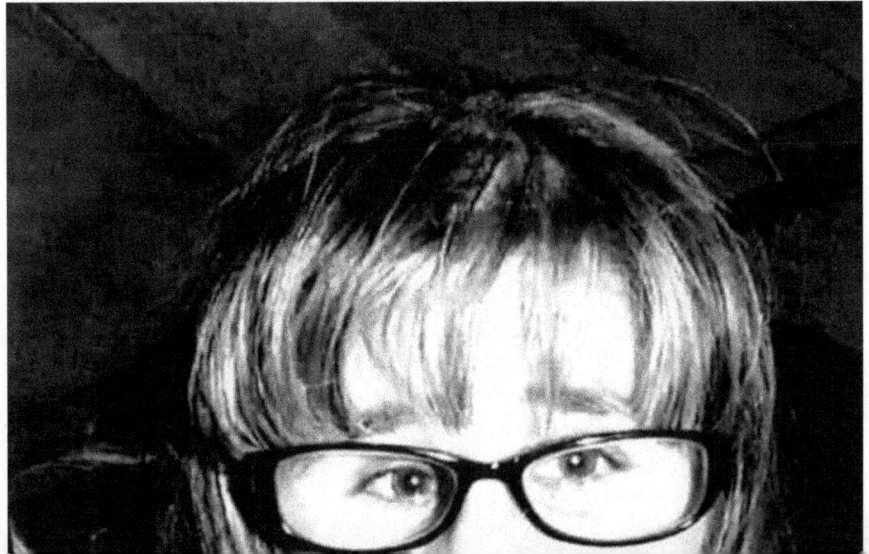

CONTENTS

Dedication   V

FOREWORD BY DR SHEHLA MOHAMMED, MD, FRCP   1

PROLOGUE   5

INTRODUCTION   7

CHAPTER 1: SIGNS OF COCKAYNE IN PREGNANCY   11

CHAPTER 2: ENTER AMY!   18

CHAPTER 3: FEEDING   25

CHAPTER 4: AMY SYNDROME?   32

CHAPTER 5: NOT FITTING IN   39

CHAPTER 6: IS IT COCKAYNE SYNDROME?   45

CHAPTER 7: SIBLINGS!   53

CHAPTER 8: TREMORS   60

CHAPTER 9: A MORE HOLISTIC APPROACH   68

CHAPTER 10: A DIAGNOSIS!   74

CHAPTER 11: THE START OF AMY AND FRIENDS   80

CHAPTER 12: IT'S COCKAYNE NOT COCAINE!	90
CHAPTER 13: DIABETES?	100
CHAPTER 14: OUR CONFERENCES	106
CHAPTER 15: THE SCIENTISTS	116
CHAPTER 16: COCKAYNE SYNDROME AS AN ADULT	129
CHAPTER 17: THE IDEA FOR A CLINIC	135
CHAPTER 18: CONSENT	145
CHAPTER 19: THE CLINIC OPENS!	152
CHAPTER 20: GOODBYE	160
CHAPTER 21: THE CLINIC	169
EPILOGUE	178
ABOUT THE AUTHOR	179

FOREWORD BY DR SHEHLA MOHAMMED, MD, FRCP

For Jayne, whose immense care and determination has changed the lives of so many families.

In writing this foreword, I have reflected on my personal and professional experience as a paediatrician and geneticist, having spent many decades caring for children with rare and complex medical conditions, including Cockayne Syndrome.

Early in my career, it became apparent that the care of such patients presented considerable challenges, not only due to the medical complexity of the condition involved but also because of the fragmented nature of existing healthcare systems. I recall the heavy burden placed on families to navigate and coordinate multiple specialists independently, leading to significant and constant emotional strain.

The advances in genetic research led to more children being diagnosed with rare conditions including Cockayne Syndrome and it soon became clear that these children required a dedicated, multidisciplinary service capable of delivering truly integrated care: a service that was not only comprehensive but one that worked with families to achieve supportive, holistic, and compassionate care.

In close collaboration with Professor Alan Lehmann and a remarkable parent advocate, Jayne Hughes, we engaged in a ten-year endeavour of discussion, debate, and dialogue to secure recognition and support from NHS England for a dedicated highly specialist service. The model of care was developed in consultation with the parents of affected children to secure an enduring and centrally funded national service.

This sustained effort culminated in the establishment of the Cockayne Syndrome and Related Disorders Clinic in London, a development that has significantly enhanced the provision of care for affected children and their families.

Now in its sixth year, the service continues to grow and evolve, shaped by the voices of children and their families, together with a highly dedicated team of clinical specialists including our irreplaceable specialist Queen's nurses, and of course the continued and unstinting commitment of Amy and Friends.

Jayne's persistence, insight, and advocacy on behalf of families was pivotal to bringing this service to fruition. Her courage and commitment describing the personal journey with her daughter Amy has developed into a powerful force for change providing hope, structure, and a sense of community for countless families.

Jayne was awarded a British Empire Medal (BEM) in the New Year Honour's List 2025, a fitting accolade for the significant contribution she has made in supporting services to children with DNA repair disorders and their families.

Her collective and collaborative approach continues to influence the landscape of rare disease care. It exemplifies the transformative potential of patient and family engagement in shaping healthcare policy and practice for patients with rare and complex conditions.

"It always seems impossible until it is done" Nelson Mandela 2001

Dr Shehla Mohammed

Consultant in Paediatric Clinical Genetics

&

National Lead for the CS/TTD Highly Specialist Service

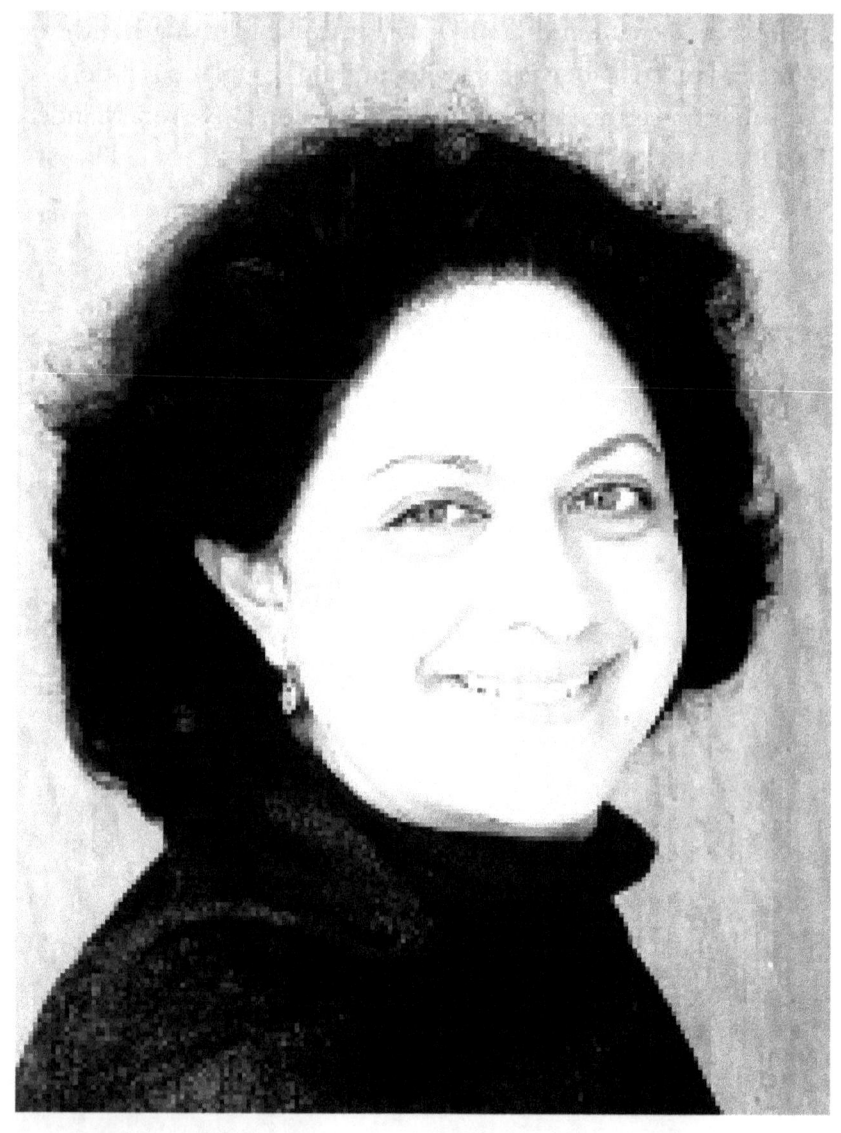

PROLOGUE

In 2010, twin girls with Cockayne Syndrome died within hours of each other in Australia. As the head of Amy and Friends, the charity for the genetic disorder, their parents contacted me immediately. The news came as a shock, but it was the final piece to the puzzle we had worked on since our daughter had been diagnosed with it.

You see, unable to find a doctor who was interested in the DNA repair disorder that is Cockayne, we turned to collecting data on it ourselves. We contacted all of the families in our charity every six months and catalogued any deterioration in the children. It is an incredibly complex illness that attacks the body in many debilitating ways. Compiling a list of all the symptoms was a massive task.

But then we found an uncomfortable pattern.

Case after case of children were dying within hours of developing extremely mild infections. The infections were varied, but one thing wasn't.

All of them had been given the same antibiotic.

Metronidazole.

We couldn't prove it, but we were sure this broad-spectrum antibiotic was behind it.

We flagged it up on our website, but without proof, we couldn't do anything else.

And then those precious twin girls died.

They'd been just a little bit under the weather. Their GP, who adored them, suspected a slight infection, perhaps a UTI. It's hard to identify exact problems with Cockayne Syndrome. So he gave them **Metronidazole**, which covers a number of things.

Their condition immediately worsened, and they were admitted into hospital where their **Metronidazole** was given to them via IV.

Within 24 hours, they were both dead.

It was a devastating blow to their parents, to their GP, and to the community of Amy and Friends.

And it was the last bit of evidence we needed.

We handed all of our findings to Dr Brian Wilson, a geneticist who was at the start of his career. With his help, it was proven, without a shadow of a doubt, that **Metronidazole shuts down the liver of people with Cockayne Syndrome within 24 hours of taking it.**

His paper was published and Amy and Friends paid to make it accessible online to everyone.

Metronidazole now contains a warning on all packets that it should not be taken by people with Cockayne.

We did that.

We ended up passing all of our collected data to Dr Wilson, with parental permission, and with him, we produced the biggest Natural History study on Cockayne Syndrome to date.

My name is Jayne Hughes.

I am a mother.

My daughter had Cockayne Syndrome.

And I have a hell of a lot to teach you about it.

Because Metronidazole is just the beginning.

INTRODUCTION

Cockayne Syndrome.
Most people have never heard of it.
They're the lucky ones.
Most people have never heard me sing, either.
They're the lucky ones, too.

Everyone who came to Amy and Friends' last conference has heard me sing Chanson d'Amour. It wasn't hugely in tune, but it was fun and an entire hall full of people, parents, families, and eminent scientists all joined in with the 'ratatatata' quite spectacularly. This was immediately after a question-and-answer session between parents and carers of children with Cockayne Syndrome and some of the world's leading scientists from multiple disciplines.

At Amy and Friends, we try to approach everything with enthusiasm, energy, and fun. But then, Amy and Friends is a little bit different; we do things our own way. You don't get to choose to have Cockayne Syndrome, but at our charity and at our clinic, we do get to choose how we treat people with it.

We specialise in helping children and young adults with the DNA repair disorder, and their families, their parents, and their siblings, too, because it has a massive impact on all of them. I should actually say 'it affects all of us', because as you know, my daughter,

Amy, had Cockayne Syndrome as well. And now here I am, with a charity that helps thousands of people worldwide. We do some amazing things, we work with some extraordinary people, and when it comes to Cockayne Syndrome, we really know our stuff.

After reading this book, you'll know your stuff too.

This book will be a guide to Cockayne Syndrome, the reality of life with it, and how it's experienced by patients and their families. However, many of the things that happen in this book have been experienced by people who have all kinds of rare genetic disorders. We will focus on Cockayne, but keep in mind that there are thousands of disorders that people struggle with every day. Think of this as a guide to helping people who are medically complex and quite exceptional, people who are strong mentally but perhaps not physically, and people who struggle at times to fit into the world around them.

Yes, it might be upsetting, it might be rage-inducing, but it'll also be funny and uplifting.

It's going to show you what to look for, how to deal with patients, and how to treat them the way we do at our specialist Cockayne Syndrome clinic. Because we're bloody good at what we do!

So, what is Cockayne Syndrome?

Well, it's a rare DNA repair disorder. It's caused by a spelling mistake in the genetic code of the ERCC6 or ERCC8 genes. Just a small thing, but it has massive connotations. Some people say it's a bit like premature aging, but this isn't quite true. It's more like premature aging has an evil twin, because this isn't a touch of arthritis and a bit of Type 2 diabetes. This is everything, all at once. I'll list the many, many problems the children have here in alphabetical order, rather like a Hollywood film does when they can't decide which actor was the most difficult to work with.

Bone abnormalities, cataracts, cerebellar ataxia, cold hands and feet, delayed development, dental anomalies, difficulty feeding, enophthalmos, gastroesophageal reflux, incontinence, increased sensitivity to sunlight, kidney problems, leukodystrophy, loss of motor skills, microcephaly, muscle atrophy, nystagmus, optic atrophy, peripheral neuropathy, pigmentary retinopathy, seizures, sensorineural hearing loss, slow pattern of growth, sunken eyes, susceptibility to infections, spasticity, thinning of the skin, tremors, and vision problems.

Now, despite it being rare, roughly affecting just two people per million, mathematically, this still means potentially there are 16,000 people around the world living with it. Here in the UK, there are 52 patients that are known to clinic but vastly more struggling to live with it if you include family members and bereaved families.

It is hard.

It is relentless.

And it is fatal.

There is no cure for Cockayne Syndrome, yet. You just have to manage each symptom as it comes along. And as you're going to see in the following pages, getting treatment for each symptom can be a constant battle that is fought between the good, the bad, and the NHS.

It's not always straightforward to diagnose, as you're going to see, but here is a link to a Cockayne Syndrome checklist on our website to help you:

https://amyandfriends.org/cs-symptoms-list/

In this book, you're going to see what the journey of someone with Cockayne looks like. I'm going to take you through the times the medical community were heroes, and the individuals who stepped forward to help our children. But I'm also going to take you through the dark times, when individuals or procedure stopped medical care from happening. And it's going to tell you all about our specialist clinic, what we do right, how to get it right, and how to learn and be open to learn all about this bloody disorder. You're also going to see how things that might have seemed small at the time, had a massive impact on Amy's medical journey. My daughter Amy was born with Cockayne Syndrome in 1991, and I set up the charity in 2007 after she was officially diagnosed. The clinic was set up by Dr Shehla Mohammed with help from Professor Alan Lehmann and me in 2019 to provide better care for children suffering from Cockayne Syndrome, children who had previously been falling between the gaps in our standard day-to-day healthcare.

My other three children, Jonathan, Ben, and Laura, and my husband Mark have all shared this journey with me. And while this book will primarily be about Amy and her journey, my family, her family, have been ever present, ever loving, ever understanding, and the best, most tight-knit little community Amy and I could have ever wished for.

So, if I haven't bombarded you with too much information already, let's make like hockey players and move the puck along to Chapter 1.

CHAPTER 1: SIGNS OF COCKAYNE IN PREGNANCY

Not all people with Cockayne Syndrome show any signs of it at birth, although Amy did. Heck, there are a rare few who don't present with it until adulthood. But then, Amy never did anything by halves.

Amy went into everything headfirst.

I've learnt a lot from my daughter, and I'd like to think people say that I go into everything headfirst too nowadays. After all, what truly is the point of doing anything by halves?

Amy's story of Cockayne Syndrome, like 25% of all people with the disorder, started before she was even born. It began during my first ultrasound.

Those of you with children no doubt know what it's like to sit in the cheerful waiting room of a maternity department. Bright posters on the wall, a few toys for parents with kids already. There's an air of restless anticipation, partly because everyone is excited to see their baby for the first time, and partly because we've all had to drink two pints of water, and it's getting hard to hold it all in.

There's a lot of shared camaraderie between pregnant women waiting for an ultrasound. It's a happy little spot in a hospital full of people who are sick, hurt, or accidentally superglued to various objects.

The maternity ward is the happy ward.

I was there with my mother as the rest of my family were working, and I remember it vividly. Rolling up my stripey sailor's jumper, flinching at the cold gel, and watching the young sonographer doing the ultrasound as she studied the computer screen that showed my baby. She started off cheerful. Then she stopped talking. Then her smile faded.

And that was the moment.

That was when I knew there was something wrong with my baby.

That one small change in her expression conveyed huge meaning.

It was devastating. I had already come to love this little person. I wanted this baby more than anything I had ever wanted before. In the end, I couldn't stand to look at the sonographer, so I turned to face the ceiling, and I cried and cried.

Eventually, she told me the ventricles in my baby's brain were dilated, and that I needed a second scan. I had no real idea what that meant for the baby, but I knew it was bad. When I walked back through the maternity ward sobbing, the other expectant mothers no longer caught my eye; they no longer smiled conspiratorially.

I was no longer one of them anymore.

The isolation from the rest of the world began then. Right from the get-go. I had to walk through the hospital past I don't know how many people, to get a second scan, one which confirmed it. There was something wrong in my daughter's brain.

Dilated ventricles in the unborn child are very often a feature in a quarter of all children with Cockayne Syndrome. Ventriculomegaly can mean a number of things, though. When it comes to foetal brain abnormalities, it's the most common, with roughly 3 in every 2,000 pregnancies.

Most children with Cockayne Syndrome present symptoms after they reach their first birthday; however, Cockayne can be a bit more like a spectrum. Everyone has it a little bit differently. Plus, a very small number of people only find out about it in early adulthood.

Back then, we didn't know my baby had Cockayne Syndrome, but that second scan confirmed that there was an issue with her little brain. We had no idea how it was going to affect her at all.

One neighbour posited that my baby girl was going to be 'mentally retarded'. This was in the 1990s, but I knew instinctively that this was absolutely no bloody way to talk about a human, let alone someone's precious little baby. And by 'instinctively' and 'immediately', I mean I honestly wanted to slap her so hard she could see last week's episode of Coronation Street.

You may or may not be pleased to know that I resisted.

And you may or may not be surprised to know that people would end up saying much, much worse throughout Amy's life. Tactlessness seems to be a malady that people become afflicted with when they are around Cockayne Syndrome, and it's going to be a continuing theme. There's a hell of a lot of it coming up in this book, and I'm not just talking about ordinary folk either; it's going to come from medical professionals too.

Show of hands, how many of you have extracted blood from the umbilical cord of a pregnant woman? Wait, if you're reading this in a public space, you don't have to raise your hand; people will stare, and you probably aren't as used to that as I am.

Foetal blood sampling is one of those areas of modern medicine that is an amazing breakthrough, while still being absolutely barbaric. Nobody enjoys it, not the patient, not the doctor, and not the baby. And when that baby has Cockayne Syndrome, it's less like finding the umbilical cord with a needle, and more like finding that damn needle in a haystack. You see, the thing about taking a blood sample from a umbilical cord is that it's a tricky process that you have to stay completely still for. And the thing about Amy was, she was never still for a second.

So this doctor, with the biggest damn needle I've ever seen in my life, was essentially attempting to harpoon my umbilical cord while Amy performed Comăneci-level gymnastics. It went on for two hours before they stopped for a break.

Utterly horrific.

I had to lie back down for another hour after that. It was so agonisingly painful and so emotionally distressing that I actually started to disassociate. I started to see this pregnant body being stabbed over and over, and I couldn't recognise it as mine. I began to get confused. Perhaps I am still there as they jam that needle into my stomach, and my life since has been a dream. Perhaps I shall wake up and find that I am still on that gurney of a bed, as the doctor comes at me another time with the needle.

I would like to skip ahead here for a moment and tell you how something as small as having a hand to hold makes such a big difference. Sometimes you have to go through brutal things. When your child has Cockayne Syndrome, you're going to see things that are agonising, physically and mentally. And here at Amy and Friends, we make sure you have someone who will hold your hand and go through it with you. It's such a small thing, but it truly makes a big difference.

We can't always make it better, we can't always take the pain away, but we can stop them from the horror of isolation. We can hold their hand. As Amy used to say, 'Look at me. I'll make you feel strong.'

I've said those very words many times while gripping someone's hand.

It's a small thing.

But sometimes the small things are monumental.

Finally, after almost four hours, the doctor managed to manoeuvre his needle around Amy's gymnastics that were so athletic it'd make Simone Biles put down her margarita and take notes, and blood was drawn.

I'd managed to grit my teeth and get through it.

It had been one of the worst moments in my life so far.

But something phenomenal was happening.

Something that would change everything.

And that was Amy.

Because even before she was born, she gave me strength.

If you know me today, perhaps what I have said so far, about breaking down at the ultrasound and disassociating during the blood draw, will have come as a surprise to you. That's because you'll know me as the strong one. The one who speaks up for families. The one that demands change. The one who stood in front of The House of Commons (as you'll see later). Well, every time I stand up for a child, or speak in front of a hall packed with people, or push for help for families dealing with Cockayne Syndrome, that's Amy. That's Amy's legacy. She was one of the strongest people I have ever met. And her strength lives on in me, and my children, my husband, and all of the clinicians and team that work with Amy and Friends.

This first show of strength occurred when I came face-to-face with the hospital again.

You see, it is easy for people in authority to take advantage of people when they are vulnerable. In a hospital, from the doctors, the specialists, the nurses, and even the receptionists, they are all in positions of authority compared to the patient. It is important for people in these positions to recognise this and to check that they don't forget their actions when disrespectful or lacking in empathy can start to resemble abuse. We will see in the next chapter how a doctor inadvertently took advantage of a vulnerable patient. Right now, however, I want to talk about my appointment with the hospital gynaecologist.

While I was pregnant, the doctor in the gynaecology department told me he needed to conduct a smear test. I didn't want to do this, there was no reason for having it done, and I wanted to wait until after the baby was born. This was already a high-risk pregnancy. It was already going in a very different direction than I had anticipated, and I didn't want to do anything at all that might have even a slight chance of making things worse.

So, I said, 'No.'

He insisted on going ahead with the smear.

And again, I said, 'No.'

This wasn't about me or my discomfort anymore; this was about keeping my baby safe.

That day, that doctor tried everything, he shouted, he ranted, he ordered, he pulled every trick a person in authority has to get me into those stirrups.

But I had Amy now.

And I said, 'No.'

You should have seen his fury. It was terrifying against the white clinical background of a hospital. But I walked out on him anyway.

Several years later, he was arrested for sexually abusing pregnant patients and was given prison time.

Couldn't have come soon enough in my opinion.

So here we tackle, for the first time but unfortunately not the last, the issue of consent and vulnerability. You're going to see them a lot in this book. I hadn't realised I had any choice about the blood draw, and truthfully, I would have done anything if it meant helping my baby. However, this didn't make me any less vulnerable.

But I refused to give consent to that obstetrician, no matter how hard he tried to bully and coerce it out of me.

Let's translate this a little bit to Cockayne Syndrome. When you deal with a patient with Cockayne Syndrome, the chances are high that they will be a child. This means that they are already vulnerable, even before you add their complex medical needs into the mix. Gaining consent from them, with care, gentleness, and patience, is vital. Not all medical procedures are painless but conducting them with love and empathy turns them into something that feels like help, instead of abuse. These children endure so much, you'll find each of them a little bastion of strength. I want you to fight side by side with them, not cause them endless distress.

CHAPTER 2: ENTER AMY!

Now, the last chapter ended a little bleakly, so I'm going to start this with a person who was fantastic. Someone who helped make what I was going through a little easier. My old boss Brian.

Throughout this book, there will be people who behave appallingly, but there are also going to be people who are fantastic. I want to call them shining stars, pinpricks of light against the night sky. But shining stars is cliché, and it doesn't feel right calling them pricks, so let's call them something else that shines in the dark.

Let's call them streetlights on a foggy road.

Brian was a streetlight.

You see, before the ultrasound, I had worked for a large insurance company; however, after it, everything came crashing to a halt. Brian called me up on a regular basis, asking me how I was, and he was a kind and sympathetic ear. Just a small thing, really, a phone call here and there, but it was a big thing to me. He made it clear that there was no pressure for me to return to work, and it was one less thing to worry about.

Brian was bloody brilliant.

There needs to be more Brians in this world.

At 28 weeks, I was in hospital. It was just a couple of days after that awful blood test, and I was half out of my mind waiting for the results of it. I was put in a bed next to a woman waiting to give birth. She told me she was going to call her baby Rudolph. I'm still not sure what the correct thing to say to that is. 'Well, I bet he'll grow up to be a guiding light?', 'I can feel his presence already?'. In the end, I settled for, 'I hope he doesn't have a red nose.' It was the best I could do in a difficult situation.

They tell me they are testing my baby's blood for Edward's Syndrome.

I have no idea what that is.

Plus, they offered me the choice of termination if it came back positive.

But after 28 weeks, with a little baby that was, at the time, practicing for the 200m front crawl and gunning for gold, I couldn't imagine losing it. I decided that whatever the hell Edward's Syndrome was, I was going to love this baby.

It was bloody hard waiting for those results. It felt like it took forever. At one point, the doctor steps into the ward, walking towards me, shaking his head, and I immediately convulse into sobs. It has to mean bad news.

When he sits by my bed, however, he tells me he's shaking his head because the results aren't in yet.

So just so you know, if you walk towards your patients shaking your head, they're going to assume the worst, right? Don't do it!

You all know, if you're reading this, that of course Amy was not born with Edward's Syndrome. What eventually happened at this moment in time was that the doctor finally returned with the test results.

Negative.

By this time, I'm amazed I wasn't dehydrated from shedding so many damn tears.

But the test was negative!

However, as the doctor thought that the placenta wasn't working properly, that the baby wasn't quite growing enough, they wanted to C-section it out. And they wanted to do it the very next day at 10 o'clock in the morning.

Well, I'm sure you all know, at 28 weeks, a baby's lungs aren't quite up and running. So I was given steroid injections, which you're going to see worked brilliantly.

I called my mum, I told her the baby was going to be okay, and I somehow found enough moisture left in my body to cry a whole bunch more of it out, while my mum sobbed on the other end of the phone.

Now, I'd like to talk about consent again, because what's going to happen next didn't happen due to any sort of ill will, but it did happen due to a certain amount of thoughtlessness. It happened due to the doctor thinking of me as an object and not really a human. It was as if I were a walking, talking incubator, because you see, they talked me into taking part in a trial, an experiment with anaesthetic during my C-section.

Looking back now, I realise I was in far too vulnerable a position, mentally and physically. Why any doctor would coerce a patient with a high-risk pregnancy into taking part in a trial C-section seems wild to me now.

If he had said it was going to be bloody horrific, I wouldn't have agreed to it.

If he had emphasised that I had a choice, that I could say no, I probably wouldn't have agreed to it.

If he had given me time to think it through, I wouldn't have flipping agreed to it.

Instead, I was on the spot, I was emotionally and physically exhausted, and I was a damn people pleaser.

So, I said yes.

Well, I'm telling you now, if I'd known what it was going to be like, I wouldn't have said yes to having a tiny human being cut out of my body as part of an anaesthetic experiment.

So, next morning, they wheel me down to the operating theatre. They anaesthetise me and start sticking pins in my stomach.

I can't feel it!

They put ice on my stomach.

I can't feel it!

Then they cut me open.

And oh my god I can bloody feel it! I can bloody feel it!

I start yelling, 'STOP, STOP! I CAN FEEL IT!'

The experiment hasn't worked. The pain is unbearable. They offer me a general anaesthetic, but...but this may be my only chance to see my baby. If it dies while I'm under, I won't be able to hold it, to tell them I love them before they pass.

So I refuse the general, they increase my anaesthetic, and they crack on with it as fast as they can.

It's an unsettling position to be in. You are the centre of attention. Well, not you, your body. Yet you are also the last one to know what is happening.

I finally hear a tiny mewling sound.

That means my baby is alive, right?

Nobody answers me.

What did I have? A boy or a girl?

Nobody answers me.

A couple of them take the placenta over to the window. It doesn't look like a placenta, you know, like something you'd see on display at your local butcher's. Something that'd be good cooked with onions and mash. Instead, it was a thin, transparent bit of membrane, with veins running through it.

No doubt it was fascinating to the gathered medical professionals in the operating theatre, but HELLO? I'm still here! I'm still on this gurney! With no idea if my baby is alright. Does it have all of its fingers and toes? I ask them desperately until finally they realise I'm in the room. Then they lay this tiny 2lb 11oz baby on me.

It's a girl.

It's Amy.

But then you knew that already.

She was a tiny, little, skinned rabbit of a thing, and she was utterly perfect. They took a photo of us, in that bloody awful room, and then they took her away, to Special Care.

My most immediate worry, that her lungs wouldn't work, hadn't come about, but I still had a whole index of fears. And while those steroids had clearly done the job, she was so small and already such a big part of my life that I worried she wouldn't make it.

They wheeled me into a bustling, bright, happy ward. The sun streamed in through the windows, but it didn't need to illuminate all the new mothers and their noisy little newborn babies. They were radiant all on their own.

I was put into a bed in the thick of it. They drew the curtains around me, the only woman without a baby by her side, and they ditched me.

It's a cruelty to everyone to sling new mothers of medically complex babies into a room full of healthy mums and newborns. For me, I was once again isolated from the rest of the world. I was isolated and vulnerable, and it was tactless of the nurses to put me in with other mothers who no doubt felt awkward next to a sobbing woman whose baby was ominously absent.

I felt that Amy could die at any minute.

She's not going to. She's going to make it out of that hospital, but I didn't know that at the time, and every time I heard footsteps beyond the curtains, I was sure it was going to be a doctor, come to tell me she hadn't made it.

On top of this, it turns out, morphine and I don't get along. I mean, God bless the stuff, but it absolutely hates me. I'm lying there, with all of the noise of the maternity ward ringing in my ears.

Babies crying.

My curtains drawn.

When suddenly the voices dim.

The room darkens.

And something, oh god, something with eerie deliberation starts to drag my leg out of the bed.

My heart starts to thump as the feeling of horror rises.

That's when I see it.

A shadow, too dark to be natural, standing at the bottom of my bed.

It slowly approaches, becoming clearer every step. Oh God, it's a monk. A monk with its hood down, radiating evil. I mean, I could feel its rage.

It despises me.

It wants to hurt me.

No.

No, wait.

It doesn't hate me. It's not actually there. It's an hallucination.

It's the flipping morphine that hates me, damn it.

By the time I was finally discovered by a nurse, I was damn near hysterical. She offered to wheel me down to Special Care so I could see Amy for myself. It was a small mercy, but I was hugely grateful. However, by this point, the morphine was showing me who was boss by making me throw up my ever-loving, just-been-cut-into, guts. It didn't deter that nurse though, she was a good 'un. She wheeled me all the way down with a sick bowl on my lap, reenacting that scene from the Exorcist.

When we get to Amy, she's having her tiny brain scanned by a doctor. He tells me, 'It could help babies like her.'

I assume, at the time, he just means premature. He doesn't explain any further.

I was once again at the centre of the drama, whilst being left totally in the dark. And of course I realise now that he was talking about it helping other babies with genetic disorders. They just didn't bother telling me.

After all, I was just her mum. I clearly wasn't important.

In case you don't know, I'm rolling my eyes right now. I'm sure you've met professionals you've rolled your eyes at, too.

Well, that was Amy and me for the next five days.

It's not the start any mother wants.

But it's the start I got.

So let's move on to the issues of caring for a baby with undiagnosed Cockayne Syndrome and how Amy and Friends helps with those problems, because Cockayne Syndrome can throw problems at you right from the starting pistol.

So without further ado,

BANG.

CHAPTER 3: FEEDING

When I finally brought Amy home, she weighed a whopping 3½lbs. She had spent nine days in three different departments, and she was doing well. It was terrifying bringing such a weenie, delicate baby home, but it was also a relief because towards the end, I was having to go home every night, and I dreaded leaving her every time.

She was strong, though. Tiny but strong. The nurse had told me she screamed louder than any of the babies in their unit. She had the lungs of an enthusiastic operatic soprano, one who was out of tune and insistent on doing encores nobody had asked for.

That's my girl.

Now, about 25% of children present symptoms of Cockayne Syndrome at this point. So this is when specialists, doctors, and clinicians nowadays might start dealing with them as patients. And here is the thing about children with Cockayne Syndrome:

It's really, really, bloody difficult to get them to eat.

They're not doing it on purpose. Their stomachs are absolutely tiny, and at the clinic we are starting to realise that it's even more complicated than that.

So, in a style that is typical for Cockayne sufferers, Amy didn't feed. She couldn't latch on, so was bottle-fed, and it was impossible to get anything more than the tiniest amounts into her.

It didn't, however, seem to bother her at all.

I mean, it bothered me. It was bloody awful for me, but she was as strong as anything. Heck, at 6 weeks old, she was hooking her little feet under the sofa and trying to use it as leverage to sit upright.

She was amazing!

She just didn't want to drink any formula.

At that moment in time, the district nurse was visiting every day with her little scales on which to weigh Amy.

I hated it.

Some days she'd gain a whole ounce! Some days she'd lost an ounce. The days she'd lost weight, I'd get scornful, judgmental looks from this nurse that could reduce Mike Tyson to a quivering heap.

This is something many parents of children with Cockayne go through. They get accused of starving their kids. In severe cases, they get their kids taken away from them. It is a horrifying time.

Just recently, we helped a young family whose son showed signs of Cockayne Syndrome right from birth. This baby was born with multiple conditions, cataracts, for example, something extraordinarily rare for a newborn. The hospital dealing with the child noted that there were signs of the baby having a genetic disorder; however, this didn't stop them from taking him from his mum and dad and handing him over to a foster mother when he failed to gain weight. They blamed the mother for not feeding him correctly. Of course, the baby has Cockayne Syndrome; it doesn't matter who is holding the bottle; they're not going to drink much from it. Heck, Jamie Oliver himself could serve the formula, with a parsley garnish and all they'd manage is a few sips.

Babies with Cockayne Syndrome cannot physically take in very much milk at all.

So what did the hospital do when the foster mother also failed to get the baby to drink the quantity of formula they had decided was the acceptable amount?

Well, they took the baby away from the foster mother, too, and made him a ward of the hospital.

For too long this child has lived in a hospital when he should have been in his mother's arms. It's heartbreaking, especially as they knew he had a genetic disorder.

The mother got in touch with us here at Amy and Friends, and I'm overjoyed to tell you that he is now back home, where he belongs, with his loving mum, dad, and family.

So, back when Amy was a baby and I dreaded those daily weigh-ins, there had been a very real chance that they could have taken her away from me if she hadn't put on any weight. It was a fraught situation.

I started ducking down on the kitchen floor and hiding from that nurse on days when I just couldn't face her. The stress was insurmountable.

Finally, a much nicer health visitor started to call round. She was much less judgmental, and I know she was trying to be uplifting and positive when she said things like, 'I've worked with lots of preemies, they're all different! She'll catch up, don't worry!'

But I was worried.

I was out of my mind worried.

Some weeks she'd weigh 3lbs 5oz. The following she'd be 3lbs 10oz. Yet the week after that, she'd be back down to 3lbs 5oz. And so while that nurse was trying to be on my side with her optimistic comments, it actually just felt like she was dismissing my very real fears. And rather than feeling like we were a team of any sort, I just felt isolated again. I was terrified my baby was failing to thrive, and nobody was listening.

I ended up going to the GP. I thought a more medically educated opinion would help. His response? 'What are you expecting? She was only 2lb 11oz when she was born! She will catch up!'

No help whatsoever.

My fears deepened.

If coaxed, I could just about get Amy to drink 1oz over the space of an hour. I was told to feed her every three hours. It was just a desperate way to exist. She didn't sleep, she didn't eat, and I'd spend hours and hours begging her to drink just a little bit more.

I take her to the GP, again and again.

He wastes no time in making it clear that I've become a nuisance. He tells me I'm: 'an overanxious mother who just needs to give things time'.

Which, in layman's terms, pretty much means, 'p*** off.'

I honestly have no idea how I got through those dark days.

Finally, I take her to the hospital.

The doctor there took one look at Amy and gave me his professional, medical, been-in-this-job-for-decades opinion:

'It's all your fault. You're not feeding her properly.'

Blame.

They blamed me.

Despite the fact that putting a bottle into a baby's mouth isn't rocket science, he decided he would absolutely show me how it's done, in order to further cement how it's my fault she wasn't feeding.

We were given a hospital appointment where a nurse jammed a bottle into tiny, little Amy's mouth, and she pushed it right out again.

She did what any professional, caring nurse would do (not) and strapped her little arms down, forcing the bottle into her mouth. She held that bottle in her tiny, little mouth, and she helplessly choked that formula down. When it was all gone, she looked at me smugly.

And that's when Amy threw the whole lot up, right over her.

That's my girl.

Well, after that, she angrily told me to just take her home.

So, I did.

It wasn't good enough though, was it?

What a way to treat a mother and a baby!

I'm going to stop here and fast-forward 28 years to talk about our specialist NHS clinic. Getting nourishment into children with Cockayne Syndrome is a massively complex issue that needs to be approached with intelligence, delicacy, and a considerable amount of care.

Enter one of the many utterly wonderful specialists we have on hand at our clinics:

Julia Hopkins.

Julia Hopkins is a dietitian and one of the most dedicated professionals I've come across. You see, nothing is straightforward for children with Cockayne Syndrome. Even the most fundamental things, like eating, become complicated.

It doesn't matter how old the child, if they have Cockayne, they're just going to struggle with food. I've already said that one reason for this is their tiny stomachs, that are so small they can't handle a full bottle of formula. Most can't breastfeed either. At the clinic we've come to the realisation that many children with Cockayne Syndrome have underdeveloped muscles around their mouths that stop them from being able to latch on and get a proper seal. We demonstrated to professionals and parents how bloody hard this can make eating by getting them to eat and drink without fully closing their mouths.

It's beyond difficult.

It's also bloody exhausting.

And the minute you experience it; you begin to understand why it's so hard for children with Cockayne Syndrome to eat much.

And what you eat, impacts everything.

Children with Cockayne Syndrome get acid reflux. And it's like acid reflux on steroids. Their stomach acid flows up the wrong way, burning their throats and mouths, causing sores that struggle to heal, until it's vomited out onto clothing and furniture. It's so horrifyingly acidic, you can smell it, and it discolours every fabric it touches.

Anyone who's gone to bed after six pints and a chicken vindaloo will know the joys of acid reflux. Well, multiply that by a hundred.

That's what these precious little children go through.

They also go through the horrors of constipation and diarrhoea, and it's a constant battle. But it's a battle that our wonderful dietitian, Julia Hopkins, is gladiatorial at fighting.

Julia has changed everything for our kids. She really has. In fact, despite being semi-retired, she still works tirelessly in the clinic and with Amy and Friends, supporting patients with Cockayne Syndrome. She made it her mission to understand what was going so wrong in their little stomachs that medication didn't come near to helping it. So, she set to work changing formulas. Some children would have less protein in theirs, for example. She literally turned their nourishment into medicine.

At our clinic, if a child is having problems, she sorts new formulas for them to help combat their issues. You can see her at any moment during clinic, running up and down the stairs constantly, changing their formulas, phoning the children's local GP and dietitian to make sure they'll know what to do. We've had so many problems with local dietitians, you see, because the children are naturally small and don't want to eat, and that goes against nature, doesn't it? It's hard when you feel like your child is starving, and most local dietitians have never dealt with the sort of issues children with Cockayne Syndrome have, so Julia Hopkins calls them and helps them understand how to look after them.

She also stops them from force-feeding our children.

We all know nowadays that our stomach is roughly the size of our fist. Some children with Cockayne don't grow any bigger than a newborn baby; hence, a tiny stomach. So, if you force a bottle of formula into them, well, they're going to do to you what Amy did to that smug nurse 28 years ago. They're going to cover you in puke.

I would like to direct you now to some resources on our website: https://amyandfriends.org/resources/

Here, Julia Hopkins has a downloadable leaflet based on all the information she's collected from all of the families we work with. She took great care with it, working with the specialists in the clinic, running it past Guy's and St Thomas' NHS Foundation Trust, and the families of children with Cockayne. It is the most effective and most up-to-date information on diet and nutrition. It continues to change lives, and we all adore her here at Amy and Friends. Throughout this book, you're going to hear about the different professionals and different disciplines that work with our charity to improve the lives of our children. And they are all utterly wonderful.

CHAPTER 4: AMY SYNDROME?

Toddler Amy was a whirlwind. A tiny, happy, laughing little tornado. She did everything quickly, like she was living on fast-forward. Her first word was scarecrow! What happened to 'Mama'! What did I say earlier? That she never did anything by halves? Why start with 'Mama' when you can open with 'Scarecrow'? And why say it once when you can repeat it over and over and over and over...

She aced her developmental test. She did all of the tasks at lightning speed, then attempted to parkour off the filing cabinet while the nurse was talking to me.

She was just freaking adorable.

And she looked freaking adorable when I took her to Liverpool hospital one day after receiving, out of the blue, a letter for an appointment with the genetics department.

I can recall exactly how she looked: pink dungarees, pink toddler shoes, and a pink bow in her blond hair. She laughed all the way there, pulling and swinging on my arm as we walked through the hospital hallways. Her voice was little and high-pitched, like Minnie Mouse. So stinking cute.

In the waiting room, there was a rocking horse, and she clambered up faster than any of the other kids and rocked like she was winning the Grand National.

It is often characteristic of children with Cockayne Syndrome that they are sweet-natured. They're quick to laugh, outgoing, and always have a smile to offer. They have a great sense of humour and amazing resilience. In short, children with Cockayne Syndrome are some of the best human beings on the planet. They are all individuals and obviously all different, but they tend to just have the sweetest, most precious personalities.

Amy was no different. Even as a teenager, when I woke her for school, she'd open her eyes and smile and say, 'I love you, Mum.'

If you have teenagers at home, you'll know how extraordinary that is. I have three fantastic kids, as well as Amy, and they woke up in the mornings exactly the same way I did, with a grunt and occasionally the odd expletive that it couldn't possibly be morning already, could it?

There are many reasons why it's important for medical specialists who deal with children with Cockayne Syndrome to actually meet them. Face-to-face. Because you're going to love them. And it will make you so much better at what you do when you truly know who you're working for.

I had no idea what was going to happen that day at Liverpool hospital during that appointment. The letter hadn't told me, so I waited in the genetics department with my laughing, playing child until we were called in.

The doctor who saw us spent a long time staring at Amy before asking me if I'd noticed anything unusual about her.

So, I told him exactly what he could see with his own eyes, that she was small. I told him she didn't really eat, that she wasn't growing at the same rate as other children, and that she didn't fit onto any growth charts.

This constant measuring is a part of all children with Cockayne Syndrome's lives. Continual measuring, just to be told what we already know, that they're small. Amy and Friends have a whole new bespoke growth chart, which has been developed as part of an international collaboration with clinicians from around the world. It's a better and far more appropriate chart. A better chart. A chart that is specific to Cockayne Syndrome. Because there is nothing worse than being shown a growth chart by a medical professional and getting told that your child is not only too small to be on the lowest bar of the chart, that in fact they lie two inches below the sheet of paper the chart is on, right there on the desk.

What's the point of measuring children on a chart that's not suitable for them?

I'll tell you now, there's no point.

On Amy and Friends' website, you can find our specialised charts in our resources here:

https://amyandfriends.org/resources/

So, if you're dealing with a child with Cockayne Syndrome, chuck your standardised charts out the window and use our charts instead. Then you should probably climb out your window and get your chart back for your next non-Cockayne patient.

Back at the hospital, after he'd spent enough time staring at my daughter, he told her to leave the room and play with their play leader so that he could talk to me without her.

All of these moments will be etched into my memory forever. As much as you try to remember only the good things, the bad stuff persists, doesn't it?

He gave it to me really quite bluntly.

He said, 'I think she has a rare condition. A syndrome. It's likely genetic. I don't know what it is. Let's call it Amy Syndrome.'

And then,

'She'll probably have a very short life expectancy. Take her home and get on with it.'

That was it.

She probably won't live long, now take her home.

My mind was spinning. I wanted to know exactly what this genetic condition was. Amy Syndrome? What a stupid, tactless thing to say. I wanted to know. I needed to know what it really was. And I wanted to know if there was anything that could be done.

I was told nothing could be done.

I was reeling so hard, with rushing in my ears, my thoughts were jumbled and deafening. I have no idea how I stood up and walked back out to Amy. I felt like I needed to stop, to focus; I couldn't think straight.

And Amy, happy, little, laughing, all in pink Amy, asked in her beautiful, squeaky Minnie Mouse voice for cheese. She was hungry.

I stagger, a million miles away, to the hospital café and buy her a small tub of grated cheese that she eats while excitedly looking through the toys, magazines, and balloons on sale.

She's going to die.

She's going to die soon.

I drive us home, and the thought of her suffering or scared makes me honestly think for a second of driving off the flyover into the dock. Ending it all.

The only reason I didn't was the fear that I would die and she might survive, without my love, without her mum to care for her.

The parents of children with Cockayne Syndrome, they might appear strong, ready to deal with everything. Perhaps they act like a feeding tube is normal for them, that their child losing their sight or their hearing is something they are strong enough to cope with. But I know I'm not alone when I had that sudden urge to take us both out of this world rather than see her suffer.

At the Amy and Friends clinic, we make sure to take care of the mental health of the whole family. I know that it was something that I needed back then, and didn't get. It is also important not to forget the siblings of these children, their precious brothers and sisters. I have not reached the stage in my story where my other children are born, but I know that they, too, should have had their mental health cared for by professionals. We all struggle, parents and children, and we understand that only too well at Amy and Friends.

So obviously I don't, I don't drive into the docks. I bring my precious little girl home. I have to admit, I am, to an extent, disassociating a little once more. It is all too much to handle.

That night, I tucked Amy into bed, read her a story, and turned out the light. And I stood in the doorway looking over at her, and I thought: 'I hope it's quick for you as I can't bear for it to torture you.'

At that moment, I suddenly realised that I wasn't just her mum, I was now her nurse and her carer.

Not long after this, Amy started nursery, and nursery was great! It was clear by then that she was different, and they loved her for it. They'd tell me happily how she was so much faster than the other kids, how she ran and moved more quickly, and how joyful she was. Plus, the other kids adored her.

Yes! Nursery was brilliant, but the outside world, well the outside world was not as accepting. Whenever we took her out of the house, people would behave appallingly.

The staring.

Dear god, the staring.

And the comments as well.

Sometimes people say the worst stuff.

It was on an afternoon after nursery, we were eating lunch, and a kid walked over to Amy and said, 'She's got a funny face.'

And I know. I know it came from a child. But it was so damn distressing, we had to leave immediately.

You're probably thinking, 'This is just one small comment, it shouldn't be such a big thing. And it was a kid! Kids just say what they see, and anyone who's particularly short, tall, fat, thin, freckly, or say in a wheelchair has had someone's kid come over and comment bluntly on it.'

But you see, it's not just the kids.

In fact, over the years, it has mainly been the adults. Even, I need to say here, medical professionals. Take the medical professional who came to visit at clinic from abroad. Upon seeing Amy, she loudly declared that her face was deformed, that her eyes were too close together, and her ears too low down, and I had to say, 'Hold on a minute here, this is my child you're talking about.'

Even when medical professionals decide to use scientific language, such as dysmorphic, you need to know that we are going to go home and Google it, and Google is going to tell us it means ugly.

And they're not.

Sometimes our children look a little different.

But they're beautiful inside and out.

So, let's have more tact when interacting with one of the most vulnerable demographics in this country: children with disabilities.

I'm going to bring back one of those streetlights on a foggy night. Brian. Remember Brian? My brilliant boss, Brian. I called him when my maternity leave was coming to an end, and I told him I wouldn't be able to come back to work. I had to look after Amy.

And Brian, that brilliant, wonderful, shining light, whispered into the phone not to resign yet. He said that the company was going to be laying off staff. He told me to hold out until my turn came and I'd get a healthy redundancy payout.

And I did!

£6,000!

God bless Brian, and all who sailed in him!

And with that £6,000 put aside, I was able to focus on caring for my precious little girl.

CHAPTER 5: NOT FITTING IN

So, Amy starts primary school. And it's nothing like as good as her nursery. The teachers can't handle her being small, and in what feels like attempts to isolate her further, they come up with ridiculous reasons to get her out of the classroom.

It builds on the stress of not knowing what was wrong with her.

How were we going to cope when her illness progressed?

It was terrifying!

The school isolated us, the rest of the world isolated us, and even, at times, the doctors made us feel isolated.

None of it was easy.

You will know me today as a strong woman who can and has dealt with everything Cockayne throws at our precious children.

And I am.

I am a strong woman.

And I do deal with it. All of it.

But here's the question most people don't think of when they meet me. That question is:

What choice did I have?

At Amy and Friends, we understand isolation, and we take it seriously. We have an active forum where hundreds of families across the globe come together to support each other. Here in the UK, we visit families with our carers, and we do our best to make sure everyone knows that they aren't alone. If you know anyone who needs to join our community, send them straight to us here:

https://amyandfriends.org

and our supportive Facebook page:

https://www.facebook.com/amyandfriendsCockayneSyndromeandTTD

I was extremely lucky to have had Mark by my side. I felt isolated from the rest of the world, but at home we were a happy little family. Now, I mentioned Mark in the introduction; however, we've been through such a whirlwind since then that I feel I should properly introduce him. Mark is my husband and is one of those people that you can totally rely on. He's a scientist, which you'll see comes into play later on in the book, and he's an excellent dad. He also has a killer sense of humour, something Amy definitely got from him. Mark has the innate ability to weigh people up accurately, but he's open and warm and can chat to anyone. What is also helpful for Amy and Friends, is that he has no trouble standing up and talking in front of large and important audiences, and he has an indefatigable drive to help children and families with Cockayne Syndrome. His love for his kids and his family permeates everything he does.

Some at the school may not have liked Amy one bit, but Amy, little four-year-old Amy, loved school. And I don't know how you can look at a child that young, a child that was clever and affectionate, and want to get shot of them.

But her teacher did.

Her teacher wanted her the hell away from their school.

The other kids loved her. They would pick her up like a doll. However, the teacher tried to use this as an excuse to get rid of her. They said she needed to leave their school because the other kids might hurt her.

They didn't.

She was smart as a whip.

But they wanted her out.

At Sports Day, they told her she wasn't allowed to compete, claiming it was a health and safety issue.

I'm sorry, what?

By this stage, the community paediatrician had got involved, and they were wonderful. They worked hard for us, fighting the school, telling them there was no reason Amy should be kicked out.

It was lovely to have someone in our corner, someone with authority, with a bit of clout. It made a big difference to have a professional agree with us and to see them champion Amy's cause. When the school refused to listen to him, it was almost cathartic to watch him hit the same brick wall we had. Finally, someone was going through the same thing we were, someone from the medical community! Mark and I could not even begin to tell him how much we appreciated all he did for Amy.

The school, however, couldn't understand why anyone would care about Amy's needs so much. It was such an alien concept for Amy's teacher that, in the end, she decided the only reason he could possibly be motivated to help Amy was this:

'He's only helping you because he finds you attractive.'

What on earth? That wonderful community paediatrician was a kind man, and a happily married one at that. What a seed to sow! How much damage could that have caused all around, just because she was angry that he cared about something she did not?

Amy.

Then there were the phone calls.

"Hello? Amy's mum? You need to come and get her. She coughed this morning."

"I'm sorry, she coughed?"

"Yes."

"And you want me to come and get her?"

"Yes."

"Well, have any of the other kids coughed this morning?"

"Yes."

"And have you phoned all of their parents and told them to come and get their kids?"

"Um...no."

"I didn't think so."

They just couldn't seem to get their heads around the concept that Amy was just a little girl, like all the other little girls in her class. She was small, but that was it. They treated her like she didn't matter, and seemed confused that we didn't feel the same way. At one Parents Evening, I'll never forget her teacher told me that, 'Amy will never become anything like the other children. She won't do anything with her life.'

I have two axes to grind with this statement.

1. I cannot stand this concept that some people think children with disabilities are somehow 'less than' because they may not be able to work a 9-5 when they grow up. That it means they have nothing to contribute to this world. That all humans should be reduced down to their capacity to toil. We are all so much more than our ability to do a company's accounts, or clean their toilets, or answer their phones.
2. Amy, as you will see, went on to make a huge difference to the world. She helped start Amy and Friends. She motivated

everyone she met. She consoled everyone who needed it. She brought people together in a way I have never seen in my life.

So 'she won't do anything with her life' was a very small comment, but it was monumentally incorrect.

If you are able-bodied and neurotypical, if you look the same as most of the people around you, you have no idea what it's like to be different. Children with Cockayne Syndrome are like peepholes to other people's souls. The way people behave when they are around kids who look different is a glimpse into who they really are.

And unfortunately, there are a lot of rotten people out there.

I remember vividly shopping with Amy and hearing two women who passed us saying, 'Let's go round and take another look!'

Some people would just look at her with disgust. Others would come over and ask, 'Has she got something wrong with her brain?'

Their staring, and their disgusted expressions, these, I suppose, small things for them, cut Amy and me to the quick. She would ask me, 'Why are they staring at me? Don't they like me?'

It was heartbreaking.

It was so bloody heartbreaking that I stopped leaving home. I couldn't stop people from staring, but I could shelter her from it if we stayed at home.

Isolation.

It was just me, Amy, and her dad, Mark.

The rest of the world didn't feel safe.

I remember vividly, one day when Mark had arranged to meet us at a café. I tried to ignore the stares until Amy fell under the scrutiny of two old ladies on the table opposite. Finally, one of them loudly said, 'I WONDER WHAT'S WRONG WITH HER?'

I bolted.

I wrapped Amy's sandwich in a napkin, and we got out of there, back to the safety of our home.

And I know that lady hasn't spent a second thinking about her words and her behaviour that day. I know she'd consider it a small thing. But as I keep saying, sometimes the small things, sometimes the small things are the really big things.

So I ran us home.

Poor Mark! He thought he'd been stood up by his own wife and daughter!

We went out for dinner instead later that day, and Mark showed me just how he dealt with the staring people.

He strode into the pub carrying Amy, and when everyone turned and stared at her, like they usually did, he announced, 'This is my Amy! Isn't she wonderful!'

And he's right. She was! She was utterly wonderful!

CHAPTER 6: IS IT COCKAYNE SYNDROME?

Eventually, Amy's school got their way, and despite our community paediatrician's best efforts, Amy was made to leave and started going to a special needs' school. It was a lovely school, but not the right fit for Amy. Most of the children there were non-verbal, and their lessons weren't academically the right level for her.

So, when we moved, due to Mark's work, we sought out a new special school. We landed an interview at one such place, and I shall never forget the day we met with the headmaster.

He was brilliant.

He was one of those streetlights on a foggy road.

He spoke to Amy immediately, and she was about six years old at this point. The conversation went something like this:

"Aim, would you like a drink?"

"Yes, please."

"What would you like?"

"A cup of tea, please."

"A cup of tea?"

"Yes, please."

"Alright then, how do you take it?"

"With biscuits. Do you have any?"

"I do, but they're in my car."

"Well, have you got your car keys?"

And this is where the headteacher laughed in delight and chuckled all the way to his car with Amy to fetch the biscuits, while she informed him that she was going to dunk them.

He turned to me when they got back and said:

"I could do wonders with her."

And he did!

And he did!

It was a fantastic school! They understood the right way to treat children. And I would like you to now compare this to one of my many desperate, pleading visits to the GP, to try and get a diagnosis for her. One particular doctor refused to even speak to her, he just stared at her, stared at her some more, and said:

"Well, she's interesting, isn't she!"

On what planet would that be acceptable? Talk to her! Talk to her like she's the human being that she is! Don't treat her like an exhibit.

I'd like to also refer now to another doctor who declared out of nowhere that she wasn't ever going to have any friends.

What part of that is helpful?

What part of that is in any way caring?

And I'm well aware that it may seem like a small thing to you reading this, but when the headteacher spoke to Amy directly and asked her, like you'd ask anyone, if she'd like a drink, I mean, HALLELUJAH!

It's a big thing.

Now, around this time, I was about to do what every medical professional tells you not to do.

I took to the internet to find a diagnosis.

Some of you may roll your eyes at this. I can understand that you may see several people a day who have Googled themselves into obscure and half-extinct diseases, but when I looked it up, it seemed to me that there could be only one answer as to why Amy was so small.

Cockayne Syndrome.

This was the first time I had ever set eyes on those words.

Cockayne Syndrome.

There was a photo of a beautiful little girl who had the disorder on the website, and she looked so much like Amy, so completely and utterly identical, that I printed it out and showed it to the whole family. It fooled every one of them. They all thought it was a picture of Amy.

I didn't need any more convincing.

Everything seemed to fit.

Well, except the photosensitive part. Amy didn't have any issues with sunlight.

So, I went to the GP, like a freaking lamb to the slaughter, and I said, 'I think it's Cockayne Syndrome."

First, I don't think he knew what it was.

Second, he said there was no way it was Cockayne.

Now, I don't mind the first thing. Most people have never heard of Cockayne Syndrome, and like I said at the start of the book, they're the lucky ones. It's okay, I don't expect medical professionals to have memorised every single genetic disorder in the book. There are, unfortunately, far too many. Heck, I couldn't even tell you every member of Fleetwood Mac. So, that's fine. I don't mind if you have to look it up.

But the second thing? The outright denial? That was awful. It was a form of dismissal.

I wasn't listened to.

Amy wasn't cared for.

And she wasn't diagnosed with anything other than Amy Syndrome. 'Now go home.'

But from this moment on, I knew what it was. I knew it was Cockayne.

Throughout this time, Amy was happy. She had lots of friends, so the doctor who confidently told us that that wouldn't happen was wrong.

Hah!

That small, tactless, momentary statement never left me. It was one of those big things that seem small. And I was overjoyed that she proved him wrong.

She was...how best to describe her? She was always up to something. She was hilarious and cheeky. And she had such strength of character. One moment she'd be noble, the next mischievous, the next she'd be cursing like a sailor, or whoever we say curses a lot nowadays.

She was small, yes, but she was also somehow larger than life.

This isn't the most useful information for medical professionals to know, but at the same time, I feel the need to tell you who she was.

Because she was so much more than a patient.

So, humour me for a brief moment while I tell you about her as a child.

Getting her to eat was a nightmare, but she loved sweets. At Halloween, she'd tell her friends to put her at the front when trick or treating, so they'd get more sweets from adults who felt sorry for her.

She loved the neighbour's dog so much they cut an Amy-sized hole in their back garden fence for her to sneak through and play with it.

Once, when she was very young, in the middle of the night, she crept downstairs with her toy ironing board, and in a calculated move, she propped it up against the front door, and climbed up it so she could reach the lock. Once she'd unlocked it, she set off down the darkened street on a little adventure. I didn't know anything about it until 3 a.m. when a neighbour returned a giggling Amy to me, after he'd spotted her on his way to work.

We had a shop at the end of the road, and the lovely guy who owned it would give her free sweets every time she went in. It got to the point where we'd tell her to stop going in! He was giving her all of his profit! But then we'd go for walks, and when she'd pass his shop, he'd run out calling after her, 'Come in! Come in!' Because he wanted to give her more sweets.

And then there were the times when she'd stand in front of the mirror and ask me why, why was she so small? Why did she look different?

One day, when we went to the GP, I managed to convince him to test her for Cockayne Syndrome. I have no idea what I did or said differently at that appointment to make him agree to the test. Perhaps it was simply a case of persistence.

The test was quite brilliant. It had been designed by Professor Alan Lehmann and was the first test ever for Cockayne. It relied on the fact that children with Cockayne Syndrome are often photosensitive due to an inability to repair DNA that has been damaged. It was a skin fibroblast cell culture test. It's not particularly nice for the patient, as it needs a small skin biopsy from a part of the body that doesn't get to see sunlight. But it was revolutionary.

As Cockayne is a repair disorder, the biopsied skin is exposed to ultraviolet radiation, and then the cells' ability to synthesise RNA is carefully measured.

It is an excellent test. Its very existence shows that there are scientists and medical professionals out there who care about Cockayne Syndrome and the diagnosis of it, and Professor Lehmann was at the heart of it. In some circles, circles that know what they're talking about, they call him the God of DNA Repair.

Professor Lehmann works at Sussex University's MRC Cell Mutation Unit and has been a senior scientist there for 28 years. They later established The Genome Damage and Stability Centre, where he was the chairman for ten years. He's worked on DNA repair his whole career and heard about Cockayne Syndrome in the mid-1970s after working with Xeroderma Pigmentosum (XP), another disorder where damage from UV light cannot be repaired properly. This overlapped with Cockayne Syndrome, where their cells also cannot recover from damage caused by UV radiation.

So that is how the test originated.

After several years, he began to receive requests from all over the world to test cells derived from small skin biopsies.

It was a huge breakthrough.

An incredible achievement from a great mind.

However, Amy didn't have any issues with photosensitivity.

Cockayne Syndrome can be tricky. You never know which symptoms it will give you.

The one symptom she never had was sun-sensitivity.

And unfortunately, the test agreed. It came back negative.

The GP was smug when he told us the results. Now he could go back to calling it Amy Syndrome and ignoring it.

But it wasn't.

It wasn't Amy Syndrome.

Partly because there's no such thing as Amy Syndrome.

But mainly, mainly because IT WAS COCKAYNE SYNDROME – with the added bonus of another DNA disorder, even more rare called XRCC4.

Honestly, it felt a little bit like either the world around me was going nuts, or I was.

Many years later, I met Professor Lehmann, and I told him that his test had failed to diagnose Amy's condition. I said that not all children with it had a problem with UV radiation. And I said, because by then I had completely transformed into the Jayne you know today, I said to him, 'So how are you going to change it?'

And you know what he did?

He joined Amy and Friends, that's what he did. He had never met a child with Cockayne Syndrome, and he jumped at the chance to meet the kids that he had worked so hard to help. He came to our conference and was blown away by our children. He had only ever worked on cells, but now he had the chance to put faces to the cells, and he was deeply moved by it. He is now one of our most treasured scientists, and he adores the kids. He totally gets what our clinics are about. They are about caring for our patients, both medically and psychologically, in a way that is as fun as possible.

We make sure every child is excited for clinic days. It is fun, it's chaotic, it's mayhem, and it comes with some of the finest medical minds in the country.

I will never forget Professor Lehmann joining in the fun and doing a sort of Superman pose on top of our helper Meg. You know the thing, where one person lies on their back and props up the other person with their arms and legs?

Utter Bedlam.

With all of our children laughing and playing around them.

You see, at our clinics, it's never going to be good news they get. Cockayne is sadly progressive and neurodegenerative. But the kids and their families get to have fun with us. They enjoy it. It beats sitting for hours in dull hospital waiting rooms, getting more and more anxious over painful tests and even more painful results.

Because that's what we went through with Amy.

And I don't want any more kids or families to have to go through it.

No!

I want them to party, with a top geneticist doing ridiculous gymnastics on the waiting room floor.

You should have seen it!

Hilarious!

I have a video of it somewhere.

Want to see it?

https://amyandfriends.org/professor-lehmann-superman/

CHAPTER 7: SIBLINGS!

It's around this time that the dynamic changed in our house. The main instigator of this change was the arrival of Jonathan, Amy's younger brother.

It is important for anyone in the field of medicine to properly understand just how frightening it is to have a second child when your first has a rare genetic disorder. When I found myself back in the maternity ward waiting for my first ultrasound with Jonathan, I was still very, very apart from all of the other happy, expectant mothers. I wasn't in their club. I was too busy gearing myself up for bad news, again.

To this day, after four children (I'm sorry, that was a spoiler, I went on to have two more children after Jonny), to this day I have never been part of the 'mums' club'. I've never been part of a group of parents chatting outside the school gates. My access to that world has always been denied. When your first child is different, you get excluded from things like mums' groups. And then, even when you have kids that aren't different, you still don't quite manage to infiltrate any mums' groups because you have to run home to be back in time for the taxi to bring your other kid home from their special needs' school.

It's not always easy for the siblings of kids with disabilities either. I remember one lad, his brother had Cockayne, and it had caused him to lose his sight. When he brought two boys home to play, they were horrified by his blind brother. They laughed at him and then got half the school to bully him over it the next day. This kid, when his brother passed away, used to take his packed lunch to his brother's grave and eat there every day.

Heartbreaking.

So nothing is going to be normal in a household that has someone with a disability or a disorder in it.

But then, I've witnessed 'normal' from afar and I don't think I've missed much!

So, back to the ultrasound. The hospital was taking special care of me, and so it was performed by the doctor who had done Amy's cordocentesis. And I was petrified. I practically held my breath the whole time. I couldn't bear to look at the doctor's face. Until they said everything was okay.

Everything was okay!

I couldn't believe it.

'The baby's brain, the ventricles, they weren't dilated?'

'No.'

'The baby wasn't too small?'

'No.'

In fact, he was a glorious little chonker (sorry Jonny).

Now, you might expect that that'd be enough to quell any fears and that from here on everything would be dead easy. It'd be sunshine, puppy dogs' tails, and playing the baby Mozart so it'd come out a genius.

But it wasn't.

Well, no, Jonny is a bit clever, actually. He's gone into the field of medicine, and he's worked tirelessly for rare disorders.

However, the sunshine bit, that wasn't how it went.

I'm afraid I spent the pregnancy half out of my mind with worry. Until I held that baby in my own two arms, I was not going to be sure he didn't have a genetic disorder like Amy's.

I was advised that another C-section would be best. So, it was scheduled on the 26th of August, two days before Amy's birthday.

I'd like to point out here that Mark was outrageously calm during all of it. And while it didn't make my nerves any better, it was good to have a solid bit of support for all of it.

Plus, the hospital, knowing my history with Amy, was keeping a close eye on me, and I went in for ultrasound scans all the way through the pregnancy.

I kept getting told that this baby looked nothing like Amy. Amy was a skinny little thing. This baby was a pudge (sorry again, Jonny).

So, the day of the C-section came and I was a state, however the surgeon was a wonderful woman who was a friend of Mark's mum. She came into the operating theatre glammed up to the eyeballs because immediately after, she was going to rush to catch a flight to a conference.

I'm so glad she'd come in for us to do the surgery, though. She was wearing these long dangly earrings, and I joked with her, 'If you stitch me up and find you're missing an earring…'

But I'm afraid my sense of humour disappeared when they went to put the needle in my spine. It didn't matter that this time was different. This time there was no weird anaesthetic trial being experimented on me. This time I had Mark by my side. This time the baby was coming out full-term. None of it stopped me from falling into a blind panic.

Perhaps I had underestimated the level of trauma I experienced during Amy's C-section. I think most of you would agree that completely losing the ever-loving plot was, in fact, a perfectly reasonable thing to do.

And I did.

I lost the ever-loving plot.

Seeing my utter panic, the lovely surgeon said, 'I know how terrified you are. So, I'm just going to do this, pull the baby out. I'm not going to talk you through it. I'm just going to get it over and done with for you.'

This should have helped to calm me down, but I was so sure this baby was going to have a genetic disorder, I started crying harder. I started telling them there was going to be something wrong with the baby. I wanted them to leave it, just leave the baby in.

They had to get more doctors in to help, which made me panic harder, fearing that they knew something that I didn't.

It was a mess.

I was a mess.

But in the circumstances, I don't think it should be hard to see where I was coming from. I was coming from a place of complete trauma.

Well, that lovely surgeon did exactly what she said she was going to do. She got the baby out as quickly as she could. Thank bloody goodness.

And so we have Jonathan. A lovely little fat, healthy baby, who just stared up at me when they lay him on me. He was beautiful.

Mark went home to fetch Amy. He brought her to the hospital on his motorbike. She always loved the rushing wind and the sun on her face. He'd strapped her to him, and she was wearing this little helmet that was small enough to fit her because it'd been handmade for her. She came sauntering in looking like a little rock chick in it.

Mark covered her eyes, and we laid baby Jonny in her lap, and when she opened her eyes, she just adored him at first sight. She kissed him and kissed him, and sang Rockabye Baby to him. And it was wonderful.

She loved him her whole life, even when they were older and he'd snaffle her sausages out of the fridge, and she'd call him a **** for it.

She loved him.

I had a sudden fear, that Mark would love Jonny more as he was the healthy one. He must have read my mind because he told me Amy will always be beyond loved and that she would always need us.

He loved them both equally.

Not so long after we had Ben, who was also born healthy and fat (sorry Ben). He was close in age to Jonathan, but Amy loved them both dearly, and they loved her back. Finally, I had my daughter Laura, by which time Amy was a bit fed up of babies. In fact, when I told her I was pregnant, she threw the fruit pastilles she was holding onto the floor and shouted, 'NOT ANOTHER BLOODY CRYING BABY!'

That's our Amy, sweetness and light.

She added, however, 'But if it's a girl, I'll love her.'

Well, it was a girl, thank goodness, and Amy loved her to bits.

And this all sounds, I imagine, like a happy little family. Well, a big family, I suppose. And we were, we were a happy, chaotic family. But it wasn't always easy.

When you have a medically complex child, they take the lion's share of your time. I spent so much time with Amy at medical appointments, and that's not always easy for siblings. There is a phenomenon called glass child syndrome. This occurs when a child is so sick or has such severe disabilities that all of the parental focus is on them. The siblings, the healthy neurotypical siblings, feel like they're almost invisible, because their chronically ill or disabled brother or sister needs so much care that their needs don't always get a look-in.

This is an issue we take seriously at Amy and Friends. It's why we do our best to support siblings. It's why we have counsellors for siblings. And it's why we welcome them at our clinics and conferences. It's important that medical professionals understand the impact illness has on the families of these children, because it can be very, very hard for them, at every stage of Cockayne Syndrome.

I'd also like to discuss here how siblings care for their sick brothers and sisters in a way that seems to come naturally to them. They don't think twice. At this year's conference, we had a magic show that had the audience in fits of laughter. At one point, the magician invited a mum up onto the stage. She had been watching it whilst sitting next to her eldest daughter, who was in a wheelchair thanks to Cockayne. Her youngest, just a little girl of about 6, danced in the front. The second the mum left the side of her eldest daughter, her little girl moved instinctively into her mum's vacated seat and started talking gently to her big sister.

There was no hesitation.

Her mum didn't ask her to do it.

It was pure love.

Jonathan, Ben, and Laura were the best siblings Amy could have ever had. They all loved her, they all helped take care of her, and all of their lives have been shaped by her. All of them have gone into medical and caring jobs, and they all dedicate so much time to Amy and Friends, helping other families deal with Cockayne Syndrome. I am so proud of them. And I am so glad that Amy got to grow up surrounded by such loving siblings. They are truly incredible people, even, I dare say, when they are at our conference dressed up as the Spice Girls.

They've been gifts to me and Mark, and to the world, as they each strive to make it better.

So it's not been easy for them.

They have been through more than most people tackle in a lifetime.

There were times when they've been glass.

Through it all, they have been so strong.

But then again, there's that old question:

What choice did they have?

When Amy hits 11, the Cockayne Syndrome that her doctor vehemently denies she has, started to throw more symptoms at her. Her hands began to shake.

First, she couldn't do her shoelaces up.

Then she struggled to use a knife and fork.

Finally, the tremors were so bad, she couldn't lift a drink to her mouth without spilling it.

Little Ben insisted on helping her with everything, but it was clear, Amy's health had taken a downturn. One which felt like a punch to the gut.

CHAPTER 8: TREMORS

At the start of this book, I call Cockayne Syndrome 'aging's evil twin', this is because it throws everything at you all at once. Amy's tremors seemed to come on overnight, and it looked, for all intents and purposes, like Parkinson's disease.

And it ruined everything for Amy.

She couldn't do her schoolwork. She couldn't colour in or do puzzles. She couldn't do anything, and it was so awful that she said she just wanted to die. This was devastating for all of us. The kids cried their eyes out over it.

She wasn't a big complainer, Amy. She rarely moaned about anything. Me, if I've got a flipping splinter, you're going to hear about it every five minutes. If I catch my elbow on the door handle, I'm nursing it half the afternoon. Whereas Amy could be in so much pain, so much pain she could barely sit up, and all she'd say would be, 'It's f***ing killing me. My f***ing legs are like a block of ice.' And then she'd stop complaining.

She always loved colourful language!

One time I took a stray cat in, and it bit me and everyone knew about it. I imagine the people five doors down even knew about it.

But Amy just got on with it.

In fact, she was usually more concerned about other people, than herself.

So when things had become so bad that she said she wanted to die, well then you know just how awful things had got.

You might be nodding your head at this. You might be thinking, 'What an incredible person she was.' And you'd be right, but I want you to multiply those feelings by a hundred. Because she was absolutely beyond amazing in the way she cared more about other people than herself.

Listen to this:

When Amy was about 23, her disorder had progressed to the point that she was in constant, terrible pain. Her legs would get horrifically cold, and so she had a hot water bottle that never left her side. One day, when she could barely sit up in her wheelchair, when even speaking had become difficult for her, she made me stop pushing as we passed a homeless man, who was holding out a cup for money.

She asked him, "Are you cold?"

And he answered, "Yes, I'm cold."

So, she rolled down her blanket, took out her hot water bottle, and gave it to him.

When he took it, he was nearly crying. I was nearly crying. Some of you reading this might be nearly crying. It was such a selfless act of kindness.

But Amy wasn't done. She made me give her her purse. All she had was a five-pound note, which she gave him.

He didn't want to take it. He was sobbing by now, I was sobbing by now, it was an absolute scene.

She insisted, 'Please take it from me. Please take it from me.'

So he took it.

And then.

Because it was Amy.

Because it was our Aimster, she said, 'Now I don't want you to spend it on bloody drugs.'

So, when I tell you that Amy wasn't a big complainer, I want you to understand how extraordinary she was at not complaining. She was on an Olympic level of not complaining.

Take this next example:

Amy loved Take That. Later on in life, she met a Take That tribute act. They're brilliant. They loved Amy immediately and became ambassadors for Amy and Friends. They sold wristbands for our charity at their concerts, and they'd get her up on stage to sing with them. The audience adored her.

We hold a conference every year at Amy and Friends, where they often attend and perform, and at Amy's last conference, she was extremely ill. Those lovely guys were overwhelmed. Amy had changed so much due to Cockayne ravaging through her body, and they were so devastated to see her that way that it looked like they weren't going to be able to perform. So Amy, and again by this point she could hardly speak, she said to them:

"Look at me. I'll make you feel strong."

It was such an important moment, and it had such an impact on them. She did make them strong. They did get up and sing for us at that conference. And since then, I have used these words myself when helping families cope with Cockayne Syndrome. I have said it over and over, and no doubt I shall continue to say it. 'Look at me. I'll make you feel strong.'

She may have had a hard time speaking, but she always knew exactly what to say.

Those Take That guys, they couldn't quite get over how she could be more concerned for them than she was for herself.

She was like this all the time. She was acutely aware when someone was upset, and she'd go over to them to help them. Even when she couldn't walk, she'd send me over.

All this.

All this to say that when she woke up with tremors that were so bad she couldn't even feed herself and wanted to die. It meant that it had to have been utterly unbearable.

So all the energy I had spent researching Cockayne Syndrome, trying to push for a diagnosis, was then channelled into fixing this tremor. I realised that it looked very like the sort of tremors Michael J Fox had, and I became more convinced it was Parkinson's.

I went back and forth to the GP. This particular GP did listen to me, and he did care, but he needed a specialist to diagnose Amy with Parkinson's. And unfortunately, he couldn't refer her to any of them because she was just a child. Due to Parkinson's being an old person's problem, there were no specialists who would deal with its existence in a child. I can't even tell you how wildly frustrating this was, and it is something that we have rectified in our clinic.

This 'falling through the gaps' of NHS care is going to crop up several times in this book, and when you have a child who so desperately needs help, it makes you want to scream.

The GP, who could not refer us to a specialist, did the only thing he could do, he referred us to a paediatrician.

So, I found myself in front of yet another medical professional, in another clinic room, once again pleading for help.

The paediatrician didn't listen.

Didn't care.

And certainly, didn't bother diagnosing.

She was dismissing and frustrating, and the only thing she'd do was weigh and measure Amy and plot it on a chart. Then she'd schedule us to come back every three months.

That was it.

That was the sum total of her help.

And so, after going and getting Amy measured time and time again with her, when she told us once more to come back in three months, I said, 'For what? If you're just going to weigh and measure her again, we can do that at home, can't we? There's just no point. You need to refer us to someone who can help her.'

But I didn't know who she could refer us to, and she didn't know or care, either.

So I was back to where I started. Desperately Googling Michael J Fox!

I found out in one search what medication he was taking for his tremors, and I headed back to the GP and asked him to prescribe it for Amy. However, he couldn't prescribe it because he didn't know what Amy's underlying condition was, and so we went round and round, with the doctors refusing to treat her tremors, telling me I was just overanxious.

And I was!

I was overanxious.

But someone had to be!

This went on for years.

YEARS.

Throughout all of this, I was seeking help from anyone I could think of. I discovered a group called The Child Growth Foundation in America. I sent them pictures of Amy. They responded that she was clearly little, but they didn't know what they could do to help.

I was constantly reaching out for help.

And I was constantly disappointed.

There was no help for Amy, anywhere.

Nobody was even interested in helping.

It was like one of those nightmares where you're screaming and no sound comes out. It felt like it couldn't get any worse.

And then it did.

Because one morning, Amy woke up unable to use her left leg. Instead, it dragged behind her as she walked. She fell over constantly, breaking her nose because her hands wouldn't reflexively go out to save her. At the same time, her speech was starting to change, and her hearing was beginning to fade.

Cockayne was kicking in.

When her left leg started to stick out when she was sitting, with her foot turned unnaturally inwards, we were referred to one of the top orthopaedic specialists in the country.

Let's call him Dr Mottishead.

Dr Mottishead is near the front of our list of medical personnel who not only didn't help, but who actively made our lives worse.

He didn't like the look of Amy at first sight.

When she was up, lying on his examination bed, he refused to address her at all. Instead, he asked me, "What's wrong with her?"

'What's wrong with her?' Like he hadn't just watched her dragging her leg as she walked into his room.

So I said, "Tell him what's wrong with you, Amy."

She told him, "It's my hip."

He turned to me and repeated, "What's wrong with her?"

I informed him that she had just told him, then I said, "Tell him again, Amy."

And she did! She said, "It's my hip. It's hurting."

I'm sure many of you reading this will, at some point, have found yourself lying on an examination bed, needing help from a doctor. It's a vulnerable place to be, lying down while a doctor looms over you. You feel helpless.

All good doctors need to understand this and be caring, especially when a patient is particularly vulnerable. Especially when they are dealing with a disabled child.

Brave little Amy did the best to advocate for herself, but it didn't work. He still didn't listen to her. He turned to me again and asked for the third bloody time, "What's wrong with her?"

So I answered him. I said, "I don't know what you mean. She has a sore hip and her left leg is in an odd position. It raises up with her foot turned in. It seems to be happening without her realising it."

Would you like to know what his diagnosis was?

Would you like to know the diagnosis from this man, who was at the top of his field. This man who was the best help the NHS could find for Amy?

I know you want to hear it.

He told me, not her, he didn't speak to her once, he told me that she was faking it. He said it was all down to the fact that she had a poor self-image and that she was doing it for attention.

To this day, I cannot forget his words.

I did my best for Amy. I told him, "You don't know my child. She thinks she's great. And she is great!"

But no, he wouldn't have it.

He refused to believe she could like herself when she looked so different, which was an opinion that said more about him than it did her.

He was absolutely dead certain she was doing it for attention.

And he refused to refer us to a physio.

I walked out of that room with Amy, devastated. Devastated, furious, and at a loss for words.

But Amy wasn't.

Amy turned around as we left and said to him, right to his face:

"You shouldn't be called Dr Mottishead. You should be called Dr Shithead."

That's my girl.

CHAPTER 9: A MORE HOLISTIC APPROACH

After the ordeal of Dr ****head at the end of our last chapter, I'd like to talk about his counterpart. A lovely streetlight on a foggy road. Someone who listened and cared and diagnosed.

I took Amy to him because I had nowhere else to turn. The NHS wasn't helping us. So I took her to see a chiropractor.

He did something that all wonderful people begin by doing. He talked to Amy.

Flipping hallelujah!

In fact, the pair of them had a very serious, in-depth conversation about what they had for tea. Amy disapproved thoroughly of his mackerel on a bed of rice, much to his amusement. She made him go through his previous few teas until he reached one she liked the sound of.

When he asked her to climb onto the examination bed, he continued chatting to her. He didn't loom over her; he didn't make her feel vulnerable or helpless. He listened to her. He clearly cared. And he gave a diagnosis on the area that he had knowledge in.

Obviously, he didn't know about Cockayne Syndrome; he couldn't do anything about her hearing, or speech. And he couldn't really help her tremors. But he could help her with the pain in her hip.

So he did!

He told us that her SI disc was out of line, and after asking her if he could manipulate her back, he clicked it back into place.

Her relief when he did that was instant. Suddenly her hip was no longer excruciating. She still dragged her leg, but her pain was eased. The difference between this appointment and the last, with Dr ****head, was enormous, and the adjustment to her hip was only one part of that. The fact that he listened and cared, which may seem like a small thing compared to needing an actual diagnosis, was in fact a big thing to us. A very big thing.

We were getting used to medical professionals drawing a blank when it came to diagnosing Amy, but the cruelty of some doctors cut to the quick.

And it's not right.

We walked out of that chiropractor's office to pay our bill, and we felt optimistic, we felt better, and heard, and like we were actual human beings that deserved to be treated well. It was worth every penny, not that he let us pay. He wouldn't take anything from us. He was a streetlight along a road that had only been made foggier by Dr ****head.

By this stage, we'd moved house again, and we hit the jackpot a second time by finding a wonderful school for her. It was another special school, but one which was the perfect fit for her academically. They had small classes and caring and creative teachers. Amy was using a walker at this time, given to us by the NHS, and her lovely teacher would hand out stickers to reward the kids. Amy's walker was covered in them. I figured we'd explain it to the NHS later!

Her school was a little unorthodox at times, but in every single instance, it was because they were putting the children's needs first.

Such as the time they went hiking, and Amy's teacher carried her on his shoulders so she could join in. They were and still are such a joyful place. And while this is jumping forward a few years, they got her through all of her exams brilliantly. I'm going to come back to them before the end of this chapter because they're going to do something amazing for Amy. Talk about streetlights, these guys were the Blackpool illuminations.

Right, back we go. Back to the day we'd had our dreadful appointment with Dr ****head. We'd come home deeply upset and angry. I'll admit, I was furious. And so when my doorbell rang and a political canvasser stood there hoping to convince me to vote for them, I sort of exploded on her. I told her that I wasn't voting for anyone because no one cared about my child. And then I called Amy. I told this woman to stay right there, and I called Amy again.

Out came Amy, she walked to me with great difficulty. She had to hold onto the wall to get to me because she had no balance anymore. And I suppose it was cruel of me to do it, but I did. I made sure that canvasser saw just how hard everything was for Amy. Then I helped her back and confronted the canvasser again. I told her, 'No one's helping me. I don't know what to do next. I know what's wrong with her, but none of her doctors believe me.'

I directed all of my frustration onto this unwitting woman, but she took it all in, and she said she'd get in touch with the newspapers. She told me, 'They'll run your story.'

The next day, a reporter came to the house and spoke to us, and before I knew it, we'd made the front page.

The front page!

It was so shockingly unexpected, but it changed everything.

And I mean everything.

All of those people who'd stared at Amy in disgust were suddenly more understanding. Many of them came over to us and asked how they could help. Suddenly people were treating her like a human being. We had neighbours come to the house to ask what they could do. And in particular, we had the man who lived opposite us knock on our door. He said that he'd never wanted to ask what was wrong with Amy, but he had a friend who was the head of a hospital in America, and he asked if he could send him the newspaper article.

Within days, I was on the phone with a doctor who had experience with Cockayne Syndrome. I spent two hours talking to him, sending him photos and videos of Amy. His conclusion was this:

"I'm pretty sure she's got it. Can you come over to America?"

Come over to America!

I knew we had to get Amy to that hospital, but it'd cost too much.

I think this is a good time to talk a little bit about how disabilities affect families economically. My ability to work had been limited right from the very start of Amy's life, as soon as that ultrasound came back abnormal.

Children with disabilities often need round-the-clock care. Which means one parent cannot work. If your child is well enough to go to school, it frees up some time during the day, but then you still need to find a job that only needs you between 9 am and 3 pm. You need to find a job that is also okay with you ducking out three times a week to take your kid to medical appointments. Plus, they need to be happy to give you days off every time your kid is sick, or every time their disabilities overwhelm them too much to go to school. Plus, the things other parents take for granted, like breakfast clubs and out-of-school clubs, well, those things don't exist for children with disabilities. You can forget babysitters, too.

No, when your child has mental or physical disabilities, when they're medically complex?

You're on your own.

I was lucky; I had Mark, but many mothers are out there struggling along by themselves.

And it's bloody hard.

Frankly, it's still bloody hard when there are two of you. When you're a single parent, it's almost impossible. So families are reduced to just one wage earner, or no wage earners, in the case of some people. Finances are always hard. Many families have had to make the choice between heating and eating. Cockayne Syndrome often causes poor peripheral circulation; children struggling with it are often so freezing cold that it becomes painful, so families tend to choose warmth over food.

Amy and Friends tries its best to help families out who are hurting for money. During COVID, when things got even worse, we sent food and money to families that needed it. When families come to our clinic, we pay for all of their transport, for the hotel, and for all their food while they are there.

No kid with Cockayne Syndrome is going to miss out on treatment while I'm in charge. And Amy and Friends will go on helping families even when I'm not. It's what we do, and we're bloody good at it.

If you want to help us keep going, please kindly donate here: https://amyandfriends.org/donations/

So when that doctor said, 'Can you come over to America?'

I was jumping for joy one minute, while my heart sank the next. We couldn't afford it.

However, people had started sending donations to the newspaper. I hadn't known this and I certainly hadn't asked for it. My initial reaction was to refuse it, but then I realised, this could help get us to the States.

Knowing this was our aim, the teachers at Amy's school started to plot. They got together, those magnificent lunatics, and they did a sponsored skydive. And they raised the remaining amount that we needed to get Amy to America. They're just wonderful

I still speak to them regularly today, and they're ridiculously awesome human beings.

So what do you know? Thanks to all of those amazing people, we were off to Boston!

CHAPTER 10: A DIAGNOSIS!

If you don't belong to a minority, be that due to physical looks, sexuality, neurodiversity, or any number of things that make you different to everyone around you, then you'll see people just like you every day. We hear all the time how representation matters. For example, more girls aspire to be footballers or scientists when they see women's football on TV or attend lectures by women scientists.

When you have Cockayne Syndrome, nobody looks like you. You are always the odd one out. You can never feel like one of the crowd, fitting in. A lot of the time, you are made to feel different. Everyone stares at you. It is hard to explain how deeply this is felt in children and their families with Cockayne Syndrome. Even at her special school, Amy looked different.

All this is to build up to the moment we stepped into the hotel lobby in Boston.

The hotel was near the children's hospital, where all the families who were attending would stay. So we were also booked in there. We were tired after the flight. We probably didn't smell particularly great. And we didn't really know what to expect.

Well, the lobby was packed, but through the crowds we saw a face looking at Amy. We saw the face of a little girl who looked so very similar to Amy.

"Mum, she looks like me!"

This little girl came running over and just hugged her. They hugged and hugged and hugged.

I cannot begin to tell you the absolute joy of those two, of them finding someone else like them. If you could bottle that feeling, you'd be a millionaire.

It was wonderful.

It was utterly flipping wonderful to meet other kids like mine and other families like mine, who were all going through it. And pretty much everyone there looked at Amy and said, 'It's obvious she's got Cockayne Syndrome.'

So we'd not even seen a doctor yet, and my suspicions were getting validation from people who knew the disorder only too well.

That evening Amy also met Nick, a lad who, like her, had Cockayne Syndrome and who was also struggling to walk. He rolled up his sleeve and showed off his muscles to her. She was just as smitten as he was.

For once, Amy wasn't different. She finally got the chance to do normal things, like flirting, something everyone else takes for granted.

Nick and Amy went on to become sweethearts, and it was wonderful to see Amy have a companion as wonderful as that boy. His mom still comes along to our conferences, and she's the sort of person you adore at first sight. She's beautiful, yes, but her soul sort of shines right through her, and it's stunning.

Amy and Friends has given me the opportunity to meet some of the best people.

When we got in to see the doctor, before he took any tests, he said that without a shadow of a doubt that Amy had Cockayne Syndrome. He took a blood sample from her because they tested for it differently in America back then. They used a new DNA test, rather than the photosensitivity test that lovely Dr Lehmann created. It's not easy to diagnose; regular gene testing doesn't quite go deep enough. But we got our diagnosis.

It was Cockayne.

I called Mark after and let him know.

He was devastated.

He'd always been the calm, stoic one, while I had been the overanxious one. Now the tables had turned. This diagnosis gave me hope. I had known it was Cockayne for nine long years, and finally getting a diagnosis meant she might start to get better care. For Mark, however, his world had come crashing down, which frankly is also a perfectly valid response. There's no right way or wrong way to deal with a Cockayne diagnosis.

Whether you're stoic or falling apart, it's all valid.

I knew we would be returning to England soon, and the doctors there said, 'There will be children all over the world with this, there is a group in America that supports families but to access it, families from the UK, Europe, and other countries would have to travel far and wide. There and then I said, 'I'm going to find other families and I'm going to help them'.

So there we have it. After 14 years of being told I was overanxious, that I was doing everything wrong, that she just had 'Amy Syndrome', that Amy was faking it for attention, after all of it, all of that absolute rubbish, we got a diagnosis.

Amy had Cockayne Syndrome.

It was official.

I'm not the sort of person to say 'I told you so', but I think these were particularly extraordinary circumstances and I'd be perfectly within my rights to do so.

I BLOODY TOLD THEM SO!

Now, once we had the diagnosis, we were referred to Professor Peter Kang. Professor Kang is a paediatric neurologist, and he's just superb. Talk about a streetlight on a foggy night, the man is an entire lighthouse in a pea souper.

Though he worked with children with rare neurological genetic disorders, he had never met anyone with Cockayne Syndrome before. When he met Amy he was immediately interested in helping her. Professor Kang has become a much-loved and valued part of Amy and Friends, and he is brilliant with the children.

I spoke to him when I wrote this book, asking him what he'd like to say about Amy, about Amy and Friends, and our clinic, and what he wanted to tell medical professionals reading this. His answer is a testament to how much he cares about his patients and his profession.

He's a busy man, so the following comes from transcriptions of a quick informal chat I had with him:

'I feel a lot of important events happen by serendipity. Amy was referred to me by a colleague at Boston Children's Hospital. He'd evaluated Amy and thought that it'd be helpful to get a neurological assessment, so that really got the ball rolling.

I'd never met someone with Cockayne Syndrome before her. Amy had an unforgettable personality; she was incredibly charismatic. She had this great sense of humour and knew how to connect with just about everyone she met.

And she was fearless.

She showed a lot of courage. She had all of these medical complications, and through it all she just kept fighting and kept trying to keep her body going. Her willpower was amazing, even when she was dealing with complication after complication. She would be suffering and in pain, and yet she'd pull it together for the conference. She'd smile for all of the other families and was a real unifying force. And so, she was really unforgettable. A very special patient that I had. I do regard it as a privilege that I was her doctor for a while.

If there's something I'd like to say to clinicians, it's this: We are living in a new age, in medicine, especially for rare diseases. Not only are there new therapies being discovered for many rare diseases; it's a lot easier for families to do their own research, which is a good thing!

Don't be afraid of patients who've done their own research. There could be things that they've looked up that you're not aware of. I think it's good for clinicians to try to do their own research as much as possible and be prepared if there's a patient with a rare disease they've never seen before. But no matter how much you prepare, they're the ones living with the disease, and the reason why they're coming in to see you is for guidance based on your overall medical experience.

Even if you've never seen a patient with Cockayne Syndrome, you will have probably seen someone with similar issues in various combinations. So, there's a lot that clinicians can bring to the table regardless of their previous experience.

I think the relationship between doctor and patient has evolved a lot since I started out more than two decades ago. It was still fairly hierarchical back then, where the doctor was supposed to know everything. But the internet changed how we interact with patients. Information became more accessible to more people. I think that most physicians are now comfortable with patients coming into their clinics armed with a lot of information.

It's not totally clear-cut, though. Material on the internet is often not curated, and there will be all kinds of information out there, some of it conflicting, some more accurate than others. So, one job of the clinician is to help patients interpret and filter that information. That's something that I do, and I'm open to new ideas. If a patient or family member brings up an idea I've never heard about, I'll think it over; I won't dismiss it. In the end, I might not agree with it, and I'll let them know if I think a new treatment isn't the right thing for them. However, sometimes they'll come up with something that's worth a try, and I try to make decisions that are in the best interest of the patient.

So, it's important for clinicians to recognise how the relationship with patients and families has evolved over the years. If anything, we're playing a more important role than ever but that role has changed and will continue to change.

It's also worth saying that giving a patient a diagnosis of a rare genetic disorder is hard. I've had families who've had bad experiences when getting a diagnosis. It often helps to provide the family an opportunity to have another appointment in the near future when they will often have many more questions.

It can take time for patients and their families to absorb all the information about a rare disorder.'

See, I told you you were going to love him.

We're going to hear more from him later. But for now, we're going to conclude the chapter with this:

We have a diagnosis.

We've been listened to.

We've found people who care.

Flipping hallelujah!

CHAPTER 11: THE START OF AMY AND FRIENDS

So, we fly home and everything has changed, while at the same time, everything's the same.

Amy is still Amy.

Her genetic disorder is still causing the same problems.

However, Mark is experiencing a kind of anticipatory grief that is destroying him. It is something I went through 12 years ago, when that doctor told me she'd probably die young.

Does that mean I'd come to terms with it?

Probably not. Is it possible to ever come to terms with the knowledge that your child won't live very long? I don't think it is. But there are coping strategies. Learning to live in the moment and learning to take joy from the small things. Because after all, the small things are the big things.

At our clinic, we have anticipatory grief counsellors who help families prepare for the hardest moments of their lives. And it makes a huge difference. I wish we had had something like that back then. Mark needed it when we got back, and I had needed it right from when I was told she was going to die young. Instead, I was told to go home and get on with it. And unfortunately, once we landed back in the UK, we did all simply have to get on with it.

This diagnosis changed things for me in several ways, though, because this is when I set up Amy and Friends as a support group for everyone going through Cockayne Syndrome like us.

When I say, 'I set up Amy and Friends', it sounds easy, doesn't it! The truth is, it took time, and I had help.

The first bit of help was from Dad. He was the chairman of a bowling club, and they had a committee set up for quite a few clubs. They helped me get all the paperwork sorted, and they wrote off to the Charity Commission with it. I wrote all the sections that needed to talk about Cockayne Syndrome, but they were the paperwork people.

Then, as soon as we got a registered number, somebody from the Dockers' Club in Liverpool contacted me. They'd read about Amy, and they wanted to help. So they created the initial website and let me work from their club.

Here's how it looks today:

https://amyandfriends.org/

While our website was attracting people globally, I worked on finding families within the UK. I created leaflets and sent them out to geneticists across the country with a picture of Amy on them. I wrote saying 'Amy's got Cockayne Syndrome. If you have any children who look like Amy in your clinics, diagnosed or undiagnosed, please give them a leaflet so they can find us, and we will help support them.'

We then went on Facebook and used other social media to draw attention to ourselves, and voila!

Here we are:

https://www.facebook.com/amyandfriendsCockayneSyndromeandTTD

We're on the 'gram:
https://www.instagram.com/amyandfriends_cs_ttd/
We're on whatever we're supposed to call this place now:
https://x.com/AmyandFriends
Want videos? We're on YouTube:
https://www.youtube.com/@AmyandFriendsWorldwide
Were those videos too long?
We're on TikTok:
https://www.tiktok.com/@amyandfriendstiktok
Want your social media to wear a suit? We're here too:
https://www.linkedin.com/company/amyandfriends/posts/?feedView=all

I'd just like to take a second here to point out how our Amy used to bring people together. Here, she brought people together to help create Amy and Friends, which in itself is a charity that brings people together.

When Professor Kang called her a unifying force, he hit the nail square on the head.

It wasn't just setting up the charity that made life different for us; when we got back from America, things changed for us financially. Getting a diagnosis of Cockayne Syndrome meant we were able to receive a higher band of disability allowance. This made a huge difference to our lives.

There are a lot of families out there, living with Cockayne Syndrome, who are hesitant to claim disability allowance. If you have the chance to urge people to apply for it, please do. Caring for someone with such complex medical needs makes working a normal job out of the question. Even the smartest, most business astute people struggle to make money while looking after a child who has so many hospital appointments, who has to take so much time off school due to illness, and who needs constant care. It can be hard sometimes for people who have been financially independent to get used to the idea that their child absolutely deserves disability allowance, and they are entitled to carer's benefit. So a wise word from a clinician on it would go a long way.

On top of being in a better place economically, the official diagnosis of Cockayne Syndrome meant the NHS ramped up its care. This was a blessing and a curse. It meant that Amy had two or three hospital appointments a week, but it also felt like we spent half our lives sitting in hospital waiting rooms.

You might be thinking now, what are you complaining about? You have spent the last ten chapters desperately trying to get the NHS to help you! Now you're moaning about spending three days a week waiting around hospitals!

I can understand if you feel this way.

And it possibly doesn't seem like a big thing to you.

But Amy was just a kid.

We already knew she didn't have a lot of time left. So it felt like a big thing to spend so much of that time staring at turquoise-painted walls while sitting on plastic chairs, attempting to play I Spy when the only things to look at are information leaflets about haemorrhoids and faded potato-stamping artwork done by inpatients four years ago.

I Spy with my little eye, something beginning with P.

Is it piles again?

Yes. It's piles. It's always piles.

An added frustration is that none of the departments seemed to be able to speak to each other, and nobody we saw appeared to have ever heard of Cockayne Syndrome. This meant that nobody could see any previous test results from different departments, and that we seemed to spend every appointment going over again just what Cockayne Syndrome was. Mark remembers those appointments as

15 minutes explaining what Cockayne was, and then five minutes arranging the next appointment.

These were the better appointments.

The worst appointments were absolutely wild.

You see, rather than admit to not knowing what Cockayne Syndrome was, a horrifying number of clinicians decided to take a flying guess at it.

This is how the parents of children with Cockayne Syndrome find themselves being lectured by clinicians for making their child sick by taking cocaine while pregnant.

I cannot tell you how many clinicians have accused me of causing Amy's disabilities by having a cocaine habit.

At this moment in writing this book, I paused to ask in the Amy and Friends forum if any other mothers had been shouted at by medical personnel for taking cocaine.

The answers were unanimous.

Yes.

Every mother has been taken to task by a clinician who has confused the words Cockayne and cocaine.

I'd like to linger on the audacity here, for someone to invent a whole diagnosis in their heads, rather than admit to a patient that they don't know what it is.

It's also suggestive of them not reading the patient's notes at all, as Cockayne doesn't remotely look like cocaine. So you couldn't mistake it by reading it. Which leaves only one possibility, that a receptionist has handed over the file while telling them it's Cockayne. Perhaps they've pronounced it incorrectly. Perhaps to some people it sounds almost similar. But that clinician has then gone into that appointment armed only with the receptionist's comment and let loose.

Really, the self-assuredness those particular clinicians display is breathtaking. If they had said, during the appointment, 'Hang on, let me just look up Cockayne Syndrome.' It would have been alright. We were used to explaining to people what it was. But inventing a disorder in their own mind? Taking a wild stab in the dark?

Ridiculous!

Who knows what patients with other disorders get told? Do people with Charcot-Marie-Tooth disease get transferred to the dental department instead of neurology?

Do they accuse people with Klein-Levin Syndrome of wearing too tight underpants?

Honestly!

Ridiculous.

And to speak again about blame, instantly blaming the mothers for their children's disorder, right from the start of the appointment, is distressing. Even when we know it's utter rubbish, it's deeply upsetting.

I'd also like to state here, as an aside, that if a mother does take cocaine while pregnant, if it does impact her baby, how is yelling at her in an appointment with her now teenage child going to change or help anything?

Hmmm?

Perhaps we need to wonder if it simply makes the clinician feel good, and that's why they do it.

Because it certainly doesn't improve anything for the patients.

My son Ben, when asked if he'd like to add anything to this book, said, 'Take your time with patients, and think before you speak.'

And he's right!

You can also see, from my little rant, that Amy and Friends connects families with each other. If anyone has a question like:

'Has anyone else been lectured for taking cocaine in a medical appointment?'

You'll get families from all over the world responding immediately. All sharing their experiences of absolute divvies who've confused Cockayne with cocaine.

Your question can be anything, medical or social. If you want to complain about how quickly your bathroom grouting turned grey, you'll find a few hundred people ready to commiserate, recommend baking soda, or show you pictures of their own off-coloured grouting.

Grouting. It's the bane of my life. Someone needs to invent lino for walls.

So, yes, we were getting to see more clinicians since Amy's diagnosis. I wouldn't say our lives were entirely improved by it. The NHS works very well for many people, but it struggled when it came to people with Cockayne Syndrome.

There may be some of you now remembering my faintly impertinent question to the wonderful Professor Lehmann. Perhaps you are thinking of asking me that very question. So let's do it.

'So Jayne, how are you going to change it?'

Well, I'll tell you how I changed it. I set up a clinic where children and their families can come for a one-stop-shop type of medical service (Dr Mohammed hates that phrase!). We have all the clinicians under one roof twice a month. Neurologists, geneticists, dietitians, dermatologists, dentists, paediatricians, psychologists, nurses, scientists, microbiologists, molecular pathologists, biologists, occupational therapists, physiotherapists, and counsellors.

The waiting room isn't potato art and haemorrhoid leaflets, it's arts and crafts and toys. It's where we socialise with other children and families. We have so much fun that kids and their families actually look forward to coming to the clinic. Heck, half the time they don't want to go home after!

Let that sink in.

Children actually enjoy coming in.

I'm pretty sure I could go onto the Amy and Friends chat and be told unanimously how much they all used to dread hospital appointments. So, it's really important to us to make sure our clinic is a happy, fun, and positive place.

You might, at this point, be feeling a little defensive. You might be saying to yourself that it'd be great to be able to work like that, but within the NHS there isn't the budget. And you're right. It's not your fault if your waiting room is boring and you only have eight minutes for each patient. It's absolutely not your fault. I bet there are days when you are enormously frustrated, particularly when you can't access your patent's files because a different department or location has them.

We were fed up with starting from scratch every time we spoke to a clinician, but we understood why. And as long as you were kind and listened to us, and of course didn't accuse me of being some sort of crack whore, we really appreciated everything you did for us.

What is interesting to note here is that by seeing all of these children in our clinic, we save the NHS four million pounds. I followed six families around for ten months of appointments and converted that into monetary terms to reach that figure. It was important when it came to getting the specialist funding for our clinic.

We schedule all appointments on the same day at our clinic. In the NHS, the same level of care would mean multiple appointments in each department, getting bounced to and from clinics, repeating tests, with information being lost, sometimes within the same department, or not communicated at all. Our clinics whittle all of this down to one day.

The next thing our clinic does that really makes a huge difference is that at the end of each clinic day, our specialists all come together to discuss each patient. They formulate a multidisciplinary management plan, moving ahead with each kid. A bespoke multidisciplinary report that is collated for each child alongside all the test results, shared with the parents, GP, and local care teams. Then, they contact the local services for each patient to tell them what they need.

Communication. Communication. Communication!

This is vital. Within the NHS, often different departments have no way of properly communicating with each other. Then, in places like Cheshire, there can be crossovers in location. Sometimes your clinic will be in Wales, sometimes Merseyside, sometimes Cheshire West. Due to them being under separate jurisdictions, communications can be hampered even further. It can be a pain in the bum at the best of times, but when your kid has something as distressing as Cockayne Syndrome, it can be downright harrowing.

So if you meet with a patient, and wonder if it is a rare genetic condition, want to find out more and link with other clinicians, contact us here:

https://amyandfriends.org/contact/

It was roughly around this time that Amy's diagnosis got very real for Amy, too. Struggling through all of her symptoms became almost the norm for her, despite how cruel and unfair it was. However, she suddenly realised that her future wasn't going to look anything like she had hoped. When I tell you this, I mean, at the age of 17, she woke up one morning distraught because she realised she could never have children of her own.

I was out there doing my best to stay stoic in the face of each physical deterioration she suffered, but this was something else. This was a sort of heartrending pain that I hadn't prepared for, and it hit Amy hard. She'd always wanted a baby; she talked about it nonstop as a child, and she would have been a wonderful and caring mum. I hated seeing her come to this realisation that her disabilities would not only stop her from conceiving but would stop her from being able to pick up and care for a baby, too.

We ended up buying her one of those realistic newborn dolls, and she cared for it and carried it with her everywhere. It was very like the way dementia patients get comfort from holding and caring for dolls, and it was beautiful, it was moving, and it absolutely broke me.

CHAPTER 12: IT'S COCKAYNE NOT COCAINE!

Last chapter touched on the frequency with which people, even medical personnel, confuse Cockayne with cocaine. This became such a common occurrence that I felt that it warranted more of a discussion, and it ties very neatly in with the next stage of Amy's life.

When Amy and Friends became a registered charity, we applied for and received some grants, which we used to support the children and families that we looked after. There was one particular grant that I went to pick up. As they handed me the cheque, which we were immensely grateful for, they said to me:

'We don't normally support organisations that take drugs.'

Ugh.

There are two points that need to be made here:

1. The idea that they were giving a grant for something they'd done no research on, that they had no clue about, is wild. Had they even read our application for it? Because I know for sure that I wrote Cockayne, not cocaine.

2. The thought that they'd begrudge children who have disabilities due to their mother taking drugs while pregnant is horribly callous. They think children should have to shoulder the blame and any ire they feel due to their parents' behaviour. I'd also like to say that drug addiction is an enormously complicated thing. No parent takes drugs specifically to harm their baby. It's not a simple case of a mother choosing to give their child disabilities. A little compassion is needed here.

A little compassion is needed everywhere!

If you'd like to donate money to Amy and Friends, with or without the ludicrous drug lecture, you can do so here:

https://amyandfriends.org/donations/

The next confusion over Cockayne and cocaine came from the anaesthetist who was about to prepare my daughter to have a tumour cut out of her head!

Now, the path leading up to discovering Amy had a brain tumour was absolutely fraught. I realised there was something wrong because Amy was deteriorating. Plus, I knew that Cockayne Syndrome could cause demyelination of the nerves in the brain and calcification. This was my main fear when I took Amy to ask a neurologist we'd never seen before if he could refer her for an MRI to look for it.

Amy was extremely agitated about it, which is a perfectly natural response, one perhaps that was further exasperated by the potential issues in her brain. She couldn't cope with being part of discussions about it, and as this appointment was to simply get an appointment for an MRI, I let her bring a friend to help keep her calm. My plan was to let her leave the room with her mate when the conversation became too much for her to handle.

We went into the appointment so the doctor could see Amy for himself, and then I told him, "Talking about her issues has started to make her really upset, so if it's okay, now you've seen her, she can go and get a cuppa while I speak to you."

He answered, "No, that's not okay. That's not okay. That's not the practice.'

Amy was already starting to panic, which is why I said, "Well, it is this time."

He bypassed me and stared at Amy, "What's wrong with you, Amy?"

Amy shut down. She started repeating over and over, "Mum, Mum, Mum, Mum..."

As her panic escalated, I told him, "Obviously, you've got the notes, you know that she's got Cockayne Syndrome. Her walking is affected, her speech is getting more and more affected, and she gets really stressed out listening to all of this. So she's going to go for a cup of tea with her friend."

Amy was halfway up the wall with fear at this point.

But this doctor wasn't going to help. Instead, he pushed at her again, "She's not leaving! Tell me what's wrong with you Amy!"

She started shaking hard. It was devastating to see. So, I said to her friend, "Take her for a cup of tea."

And they left.

The neurologist was furious. Whether it was because he wasn't used to things not being done 'his way', or he didn't like a woman standing up for her daughter, or for some other impractical issues with hierarchy that Professor Kang touched on briefly in a previous chapter.

This doctor was taking this appointment as some sort of personal slight rather than a mother trying to make reasonable accommodations for her daughter, who was potentially nearing the end of her very young life.

I hadn't gone in there to be difficult.

I hadn't gone in for a fight.

But this doctor was acting like I'd insulted his parking skills!

So, he used a tried and tested technique that has been utilised by male doctors against women for centuries. He suggested I was being irrational and hysterical.

He said, "I'm booking her and you in to see a psychologist. And you need it more than her!"

Actually, everyone could benefit from a psychologist from time to time. This doctor certainly needed help with his hair-trigger anger issues. I hope he never experiences what it's like as a parent to have a child that is so very ill, with something that has no cure, that will end in death. I hope he never experiences the absolute desperation and panic you feel when your child is in agony, physically and psychologically. Because it is a level of trauma that is so profound and unending that I still live with it today. When I remember Amy's hardest moments, when I remember her passing, it is torture. It was torture then. It is torture now. It never dulls.

I hope he never has to experience it.

I hope none of you ever have to experience it.

But I think there is nothing psychologically unhealthy about a mother not wanting to put her child under any more duress than is absolutely necessary. He saw Amy, and he knew she had Cockayne Syndrome. He should have been well aware of the effects it can and usually does have on the brain. All I wanted was a referral for an MRI without making Amy sit through a discussion about her brain deteriorating.

After all, your brain is who you are, isn't it!

Amy had taken her increasing pain and lack of mobility with sadness and stoicism. But the possibility of losing herself, of losing brain function, was terrifying.

This whole appointment could have been so much better.

He told me he was going to book her into the incontinence clinic and seizure clinic, because she was going to need them.

So, I said, "Thank you for that. And now, can you tell me that you're going to do the MRI?"

He opened up her file, read it, then grimaced and said, "I see you've been to America, lining fat, rich American pockets. All they're doing is research, you know. They're not going to help her in any way."

What on earth has that got to do with granting a child, whose brain function is rapidly deteriorating, an MRI scan?

I'm starting to wonder, from my vantage point years later, if he wasn't the one getting irrational and hysterical?

I told him that the American clinic had already helped her and that I supported all research into Cockayne Syndrome. Medicine cannot progress without research, right? There's a reason we're not all keeling over with smallpox.

I've already introduced you to Professor Kang from the Boston Children's Hospital. At no point does he view his patients as anything other than children, than human beings. He's compiling research to try and help us, not to experiment on us, and empathy saturates everything he does.

This neurologist, however, just got angrier and angrier. His professionalism wasn't just gone, it had flown out of the window and shat on someone's car.

He wrote the referral for Amy's MRI on a piece of yellow paper and then, instead of handing it to me, he threw it on the floor, forcing me to bend down and pick it up.

At that point, the nurse who had been in attendance was so mortified by his behaviour that she walked out of the room.

I stepped out too. I waited until he was no longer in earshot, and I cried. And Amy, poor Amy was so worried about me that I had to pull myself together sharpish, so as not to cause her any further distress.

It is just typical of Amy to be worried about me, more than herself. She spent so much of her life comforting people who were upset for her. She was extraordinary. And if I had to bend before a thousand doctors to pick up papers that they've thrown on the floor in anger, I would. I would absolutely bend a thousand times. And a thousand times more.

As would any parent of a critically ill child.

That neurologist that day decided that he'd not done enough harm, however. So, he decided to call up our GP and tell her this:

'If Mum insists on taking Amy to America, then I will not see them again. Do not send them again.'

When our GP reported this back to us, I informed her that I would take my child to anyone in the world who had a specialism in Cockayne Syndrome, and I'm sure she'd do the same!

She agreed. Of course she'd do the same! But she repeated that the neurologist said he'd refuse to see Amy if I took her across the pond again.

I suppose that was a win-win situation then, because I didn't ever, and still do not ever want to see that man again.

There may be times when you are dealing with a patient who has Cockayne Syndrome and is an adult. Please speak to them, don't talk over their heads to their carer while ignoring them. However, if they need their parent or carer to advocate for them, please accept that too!

I mean, I'm sure I don't have to tell you not to get hysterical because your patient needs different accommodations from what is the norm. And I'm doubly sure none of you would throw a referral letter on the floor in an attempt to humiliate the person who has to pick it up.

Don't be that man.

Dr Adesoji Abiona, a community paediatrician who specialises in neurodevelopmental paediatrics, takes care of the children in our clinic. I chatted to him during a conference about how he views families that come to his appointments. The following quote comes from the transcripts of an informal conversation with him:

"I think one of the big issues is that people can become cynical. My advice is to be empathetic, be open-minded, and think, 'How can I help this family?' Put yourself in their situation. Often, when families are asking so many questions, it can seem like they're being pushy. But you have to understand that this is their loved one, this is their precious one. Move past any cynicism. Remember, this is a situation where this family is very anxious. Try to empathise with them.'

Any doctor who deals face-to-face with their patients will know about the importance of wearing many hats. It's really important too. Sometimes clinicians just wear their 'scientist hat' and this might seem like all that's needed. After all, it's professional, and you might feel also like it pushes science further. However, you also need to process any information you get and explain that information to a patient or carer in terms of genetics or neurology or nutrition or immunology.

While all of this is going on, there's one hat you mustn't forget. The hat that cares about your patient, the hat that empathises with the carers, the hat that listens. I'm not saying you have to walk a mile in their shoes, some of them may be wearing high heels. But, please do try to wear a hat that is empathetic and see where they're coming from. They may seem confrontational, or ready to stand up for their loved one. Understand that this is only because they've been fobbed off before, or abused before. A little kindness, listening to them, and doing whatever you can to help, will go a heck of a long way.

Back to the MRI. We get it done, and now it is this neurologist's chance to do even more harm, because he wrote to our GP saying that the MRI didn't show anything abnormal.

This didn't sit right and wasn't indicative of Amy's continuing deterioration, which is why I requested the MRI images to see for myself.

My request was denied.

My GP then requested them on my behalf.

He caused as much delay as he could, but finally I got my hands on a disc that contained the images. I immediately opened them up on the computer, and Mark and I found ourselves staring at what was clearly a tumour, a great white spot. You couldn't miss it. I was starting to feel like I was going round the bend.

We ended up taking Amy and her MRI results over to Boston, to Professor Kang. He checked her eyes, looked at the scan, and became suddenly very serious, telling us we were right.

She had a brain tumour.

And not only that, but she'd got scalloping of the brain. It was shrinking in on itself because the fluid had nowhere to go.

Hydrocephaly.

A brain tumour and hydrocephaly.

How could you miss that?

They say, 'Never attribute to malice that which can be adequately explained by incompetence' don't they. I think this time may be the exception.

So, Professor Kang ordered surgery immediately. He sent us back to the UK for it because it'd cost too much for us in America. He referred us back to the hospital where Amy had had her MRI, and there was a horrible moment when I thought he was sending us back to that awful neurologist. But no, thank goodness, he sent us to a different doctor. In fact, back in the UK we met two wonderful surgeons. Dr May and Dr Melucci. They were fantastic. They talked so kindly to Amy. They checked her eyes and agreed with Professor Kang that surgery was needed ASAP. They really were brilliant, they listened, they cared, and diagnosed, and they made it look so easy.

However, the anaesthetist who was preparing her walked into the room, and wait for it...

Wait for it...

He walked into the room and the first thing he said to me was:

"She wouldn't be like this if you hadn't taken cocaine."

This wasn't someone handing over a cheque without looking into who they were donating to.

This was the man who was going to anaesthetise my daughter!

I told him to go away and look at the spelling of Cockayne, then Google it and come back to me.

So, he did, and he came back and told me he was really sorry.

But that's not really good enough is it?

1. He'd not bothered to read her file before planning to cut her open.
2. He was being unnecessarily cruel to a woman with a child who had a brain tumour and clear physical disabilities that were obviously excruciating.

I've said it once and I'll keep saying it. Cockayne or Class A illegal drugs. Lecturing the mother of a teenage child helps and achieves absolutely bloody nothing.

That's why I told him I wasn't accepting his apology.

So there!

I could probably fill six books by asking all the parents of Amy and Friends for their experiences of being shouted at for taking cocaine, but to have it from the man who was about to operate on my child's brain?

Honestly.

Unfortunately, they ended up not being able to remove the tumour because it was on the thalamus. Instead, they did a third ventriculoscopy, reconstructing a new canal in her brain to take the fluid a different way around to prevent her from having a shunt.

The minute they did it, Amy could walk and talk really well again. It didn't last long, but it was wonderful for the small window while it did. It was a really big thing to her and to all of us.

We, of course, had been frantic with worry the whole time she was in surgery. We didn't know if she'd end up with long-lasting damage. But when she came round, she opened her eyes and asked for a bacon butty.

We got our Amy back!

CHAPTER 13: DIABETES?

You may have the idea that up until now, we were leading angry, miserable lives, but actually, the opposite was true. We were frustrated with the medical help we did and didn't receive, but we were a happy and faintly chaotic family. Our children were absolutely brilliant and we had a lot of fun. Christmases were utterly joyful, and we all loved each other to bits.

It's not particularly easy to take care of a child with disabilities. At times, Cockayne Syndrome made life miserable for Amy, and that's devastating for a parent or a sibling to watch, but overall, we knew to find happiness in the small things.

Which, by now, we all know are really the big things.

Amy loved to go shopping. She loved buying knickers with cartoon characters on. She loved going out for lunch. And she adored her brothers and her sister.

Her mobility had taken a massive hit, but she was still a force of nature and she carried herself with strength, dignity, and utterly glorious bald-faced cheek.

The village where we lived grew to know her and love her, too. When we walked into the pub, everyone would be pleased to see her, and in a way, she brought the community together there, too. Nobody brought folk together like she did. This is another one of her legacies, as Amy and Friends continues to bring people together.

Amy had so many friends, too. One of them was Billy Hui, the Radio Merseyside presenter. He is an ambassador now for Amy and Friends, and he's brilliant at it. What gave Amy particular joy, however, was the choir he set up, called SingMe Merseyside. She adored listening to them, but her favourite song out of all that they sang was Hallelujah, by Leonard Cohen. To hear them sing it and to watch her face as she listened? Transcendent.

So, they were hard but incredibly happy days.

Amy also thoroughly enjoyed warbling like a cat (singing) and acting at her Emerge group every week with her wonderful friend Keith and his wife Jenn, they had the best fun and spent all of their times together laughing.

The constant appointments with the NHS were a bit hit and miss, though.

It felt like we were constantly going in, we were constantly seeing specialists, while still not really getting anywhere. I wonder now, with the benefit of hindsight, if clinicians weren't simply overwhelmed by Amy's disorder. Nobody seemed to want to help her symptoms as long as Cockayne Syndrome was the underlying diagnosis. It felt a little bit like, at times, we brought the NHS to a standstill.

With the NHS already under so much pressure, it's not hard to see how our clinic in London would go on to help take the strain off them to the tune of four million pounds.

So, where were we? Happy, struggling, and a little bit better off financially. The latter of which led us to being on television!

There's a show called Saints and Scroungers. It covers people who live off benefits, some of whom are deserving and some of whom are cheating the system. We were recommended to the people making the show by a journalist, and before you know it, we were scheduled to be the 'saints' of the episode.

The TV show presented a sensitive look at what life is like for children and families when Cockayne Syndrome is involved. They came and they visited a whole group of us from Amy and Friends at one of our conferences, and I was pleased with the kind way they went about it.

There's a reason I'm telling you about this TV show.

The reason is this, in between takes the presenter, Dominic Littlewood, who was lovely to us by the way, turned to me and said, 'I don't want to be rude, but Amy's got diabetes.'

Dominic, it turns out, has Type 1 diabetes, which he's been living with his whole life. So, when he turned to us and said, 'I don't want to be rude, but Amy's got diabetes.' It was coming from the voice of experience.

Diabetes?

Did I know she had diabetes?

No! I bloody didn't know!

We were going into hospital three times a week, having constant tests, including blood tests, and it took a TV presenter to smell her slightly almondy breath to work it out.

Clinician after clinician we'd waded through. Appointment after appointment. And nobody had thought, with all the blood they'd taken from her, to test for it.

We already know Cockayne is a repair disorder. We talked about it being a bit like aging's evil twin. Anything that is associated with old age is likely to affect a child with Cockayne. Diabetes is right up there with Parkinson's and cataracts.

How did they miss it?

How did they miss it?

They also, it later turned out, missed an underactive thyroid. Another easily diagnosed issue!

I imagine now that they missed it because Amy was under the care of so many different specialists and so many different departments, that each clinician focused on their own issue. Nobody was seeing her illness as a whole. Add in the overwhelming impact Cockayne has on a clinician viewing it for the first time, plus, the short appointment times, and I suppose in many ways I should be saying:

How could they not have missed it?

Dominic knew about diabetes because he's had a lifetime of it. He also got to spend all day with Amy, something the clinicians in the NHS couldn't do, even if they wanted to.

We have solved this for many patients with Cockayne Syndrome in our clinic. We test for everything when we take blood, just as they do at Professor Kang's clinic in Boston, and all of our departments get together to discuss each patient at the end of the day.

It's the dream.

Well, no, the dream would be to have a cure for Cockayne Syndrome.

I should instead say, it's the closest thing to a dream we can get for now.

You see, people with Cockayne Syndrome are so extraordinarily complex medically, needing such a diverse range of specialists, that it's the only way that makes even a modicum of sense.

What can you take away from this?

What if you're struggling with interdisciplinary communication?

Well, include the parents or the carers of your patient. They may look exhausted. They may not always understand complicated medical terminology, but they know what their child is going through. They live with their child's struggles every day. You can bet they can list every appointment, every symptom, and medication their child has ever had.

Communicate with the parent if you think the patient might have something, such as diabetes, that is out of your jurisdiction. Don't assume someone else has it covered. If you can refer the patient, do it. If you need the patient to head back to their GP or paediatrician with your suspicions of (in this case) diabetes, do it. The parents of children with Cockayne Syndrome understand that it is a barrage of symptoms that affects every part of them. There's a chance they'll have already noticed something is different; they just haven't realized it was medically significant.

When Amy started eating and drinking more, it felt like a positive thing. I'd spent my life worrying about how little she consumed, so watching her eat and feel hungry felt like a turn up for the books.

So I had noticed something was different.

I just hadn't realised it was due to diabetes.

If I had had an appointment with a doctor who had had the time to discuss Amy's overall condition, I'd have probably told them, 'She's finally eating and drinking more!' And it would have set alarm bells ringing for the experienced clinician.

But of course, as a parent, when you're at a neurology appointment, you focus on your child's neurological problems.

When you're visiting the radiology department, you don't talk about the extra helping of sausages she had last night.

In orthopaedics, you stick to musculoskeletal issues.

It's easy for me to say we've discovered the solution to communication problems in our Amy and Friends' clinic, because our specialists can physically come together in the same room and have the time to go over each patient's files.

With a cup of tea, I might add.

And a biscuit, Amy might have also added, were she here.

If you only have 15 minutes in an isolated department to deal with a patient who is having Parkinson's tremors, I understand that it can be difficult to know or to even wonder if anyone has noticed the patient's slightly almondy diabetic breath.

But you do have a brilliant communication tool, right in front of you. One which is interdepartmental.

The patient's carer.

So, include them in the discussions of your care. Listen to them and communicate with them. They may have been too busy looking after their medically complex child to have showered that day. They may be outrageously un-ironed. They may look like they haven't slept for a week. But they'll know every department's diagnosis so far. They'll know every medication prescribed. They'll know when something is off or different with their kid. And they'll be extremely grateful for your communication. They want to be part of the conversation about their child's health.

You may feel like rolling your eyes when parents say that they're the experts on their children. And perhaps you've dealt with some dreadful parents who have led you to that eye roll. But the parents and carers of kids with Cockayne Syndrome are the ones who witness their pain, their seizures, every time they vomit acid or blood, every time their pain becomes debilitating; the parents and the carers are the ones living it. If there's something not right with their kid, they may be able to spot it before you do, simply because they're with them 24/7.

So look at the carers as part of your team!

Talk to us!

I've spent this book talking about how important it is that you listen to us, but you can talk to us too!

CHAPTER 14: OUR CONFERENCES

I've mentioned our conferences a few times, so I think it's the right spot to tell you more about them. Once Amy and Friends was firmly established, we went about creating a yearly conference. This was an important step towards developing a clinic specifically for patients with Cockayne Syndrome and Trichothiodystrophy (TTD). We are currently also branching out towards Bloom Syndrome as well as helping some patients with MORC2 and XRCC4.

Our conferences started with just seven families in 2007 in the basement of a pub. In 2008, Professor Kang published a paper on Cockayne. Things took off. Today, we take over entire hotels, hosting hundreds of people, children, families, and scientists. And we do that with no small amount of help from Jayne O'Gorman. Jayne, on top of spelling her name fabulously, helps plan and organise our conferences, and we could not do it without her. She's had her own health problems yet still works her backside off for Amy and Friends. Jayne has cycled across countries, had us lying in gardens listening to soundbaths; this woman literally goes above and beyond, and has the BIGGEST heart! And did I mention she is bloody gorgeous too?

The reason the conferences were and are so important is because they bring patients and clinicians together. Most clinicians who deal with Cockayne Syndrome have never met a patient with it, even those at the highest levels, like Professor Lehmann before he came to us. They work in the lab and they are brilliant, but they don't work directly with the patients. Some clinicians have met one child with it. But it is only when we all come together that they can really witness what a spectrum it is, and that's vital for research.

In terms of the kids and families who come to the conferences, it's wonderful. It's a chance to meet up with the only other people on the planet who know what they're going through. We have times even where carers take the kids to a show, while the parents get a bit of respite.

Everyone looks forward to the Amy and Friends conferences, including me!

Take a look at them here:

https://amyandfriends.org/conference/

Now, before I tell you about Professor Kang's experiences with our conferences, I want to let you know that these yearly events aren't some sort of plus-sized laboratory where scientists go to stare at the kids. Our conferences are great fun for everyone. I appreciate every clinician who has any part in helping our children. I really do. But it's important to make things enjoyable, because members of Amy and Friends all have to live with this disorder. Life is short. And we need to make it as pleasant as possible for these kids and their families, who all have so much to deal with.

So, our conferences bring all the children and families together, and all interested clinicians together too, and we have fun! There is plenty of time for clinicians to do research and consult with each other, doing vital and serious work. There is also time for clinicians to meet the children, have fun, and enjoy all the activities we do there.

The conferences bring the two worlds of the patient and the scientist together. Some of the shyer clinicians stand at the edges of the hall, watching the children play with great affection. Others dance with the kids, lifting them onto their shoulders for the conga, and having a dance off!

All of them make themselves available to talk to parents. And all of them are interested in our kids, giving thoughtful and caring answers to everyone's questions. One of our dearest friends at Amy and Friends, Kathy, a woman you just want to hug on sight, lost her two precious boys, Kirby and Chad. She still attends the conference, flying across the pond to get here, meeting old friends and making new ones, and staying connected to the only people on the planet that can understand what she's been through. During her sons' lives, she never received a full diagnosis for them. Enter Dr Theil, who listened to her and has offered to test the DNA on her sons' baby teeth that she's held onto.

Try and ring your doctor for a copy of any previous test results for your child. Go ahead and give it a go. You can't even get access to your own kid's records without running through several hoops.

But at our conferences, our scientists do what they can to help. They understand how important it is for us. Offering a grieving mother the chance to get a diagnosis for her sons is a huge deal. I wonder where Kathy is right now? I think I need to hug her.

We have lots of parents and siblings of children who have passed, who continue to come to our conferences. We gather together to tell funny stories of what they got up to when they were alive, and for a moment, they live again. Nick's mum has hilarious stories of his antics, and anyone who has never met him gets to know him in those precious memories.

Our clinicians hear all of this.

So they just get it.

They really do.

And the ones who don't? Well, they're not the right fit for us. Anyone viewing our children as objects, as nothing more than a way to make their name famous, or as a way to make money, is not right for us. We only want scientists who care. We're lucky in that we have some of the finest minds in the world attending our conferences. We have Professor Lehmann and Professor Hoeijmakers, two scientists who are usually referred to as the Gods of DNA Repair. Or as we call them, Alan and Jan.

Speaking of finest minds, let's hear now from Professor Peter Kang, because he can tell you about our conferences from a clinician's point of view.

The following comes from a transcription of an informal conversation with him:

"The conferences are great, I've become a regular participant, and it's been really amazing to see what Jayne has done, getting everyone together, patients, families, scientists, and clinicians. She really helps patients feel more comfortable, and patients and families then feel more comfortable talking to doctors and scientists. It's eye-opening for the scientists in particular to get to meet these patients if they've been doing research in the lab. They might be working with mice or cell models of this disease, and they don't actually get to meet the patients on a regular basis.

Being able to come to a conference and actually see a patient who's affected by this, well, I think it really helps to make it real for them. It motivates them to do more in the lab.

Even for the clinicians who have had a patient with Cockayne Syndrome, it's so very unusual to have a single place where all of a sudden there are several dozen patients with Cockayne Syndrome all at once. And that really is an amazing opportunity for the clinicians to learn a little bit more about the patterns that you see across different ages and different forms of the disease. Everybody learns from each other. No matter what your background going into the conference is, you'll learn something. This is what keeps me going back. Plus, it's a lot of fun interacting with the families.

More recently, I've brought some team members from my research group, and we've done some research activities there, all under an IRB-approved protocol. We're trying to work on what happens to these patients in a way that's more quantifiable, so that we can figure out how to measure outcomes in a clinical trial. We've collected a lot of data over the last few years at Amy and Friends, and we're hoping to publish an article based on those experiences in the next year or so, with more to follow.

I think Amy and Friends, Jayne's work, is helping move the field forward towards more therapies. So, she's done a lot of good for this community, and I've always found it amazing how much she cares about all the other families who are affected."

He has said some lovely things there, but it's true, it's important to me, after spending so much of Amy's life running from one hospital appointment to another, that any medical research or therapy that these children attend should be fun. Children with Cockayne Syndrome are the sweetest, and their siblings are just as precious. Their brothers and sisters often grow into particularly empathetic and kind adults, and their parents are some of the most selfless people I've met. All of them are important and valued members of society. And they all deserve happiness. The weekends of our conferences are not just enjoyable; they're moments where they are seen and heard by clinicians. They are listened to. They are cared for. And they're diagnosed.

Amy's brothers and sister come along every year, and I am so bloody proud of them and how they relate and care for the families there with such natural ease. They have grown into wonderful human beings who are changing the world with their compassion. I love them to pieces. You can't get them off the karaoke machine, and I'm not sure about Ben's legs in his Ginger Spice mini dress, but they're bloody brilliant.

Now, for the last ten years, roughly, we have had a brilliant doctor from the Netherlands attend our conferences. Dr Arjan Theil. He works in a clinic like ours in Rotterdam, and it's going really well.

Take a look:

https://amyandfriends.nl/

Dr Theil has been doing research on the DNA repair mechanism that is affected in children with Cockayne Syndrome, as well as Trichothiodystrophy, a similar repair disorder that Amy and Friends also helps with.

You can find out more about TTD here:

https://amyandfriends.org/about-ttd/

and we have TTD Symptoms list here:

https://amyandfriends.org/ttd-symptoms-list/

Let's hear directly from him, again it comes from a transcript of an informal conversation:

"If you have a defect in the DNA repair pathway, you can either have cancer-prone features, or you can get what you see in Cockayne Syndrome children. It's the aging phenotype, and we've been researching it for many years. We got involved with Amy and Friends while I was working in the lab. I'd never worked directly with patients with Cockayne Syndrome, and so coming to an Amy and Friends conference was the first time I'd had a chance to meet anyone with the disorder.

It was a very warm welcome!

All of the families were together in the dining room, and one of the things that is very typical for children with Cockayne Syndrome, as well as Trichothiodystrophy, is that they're very open and friendly. I'm a big guy, but suddenly there were two children just walking up to me with their hands held out to me, wanting to interact with me."

It's clear that Dr Theil was won over instantly by the sweet kids in Amy and Friends. I'm glad he felt like we gave him a warm welcome, because it is exactly our intention to be a fun, safe, and warm place for all of our families. It should feel like coming home. And it particularly pleased me that he understood instantly how fun and sweet-natured children with Cockayne are. They're utterly precious.

Dr Theil then goes on to remark on the sensory-seeking nature of our children. Because they don't seem to be susceptible to sensory overload, instead the louder, the brighter, the more entertaining, the happier they are.

I think due to the debilitating nature of Cockayne, he was worried he was going to walk into a room full of miserable people, all sitting around glumly. Instead, our chaotic, hilarious antics really impressed him.

He also emphasises the scientific side of our conferences, and how it's a place for scientists to share knowledge and collect data. They also get the chance to speak to the families to explain their research in layman's terms, so the people affected can understand their findings and their progress.

He laments, at times, the lack of funding holding them back, but he makes an interesting point when he suggests researching treatment for children with Cockayne Syndrome could actually be further reaching:

"Cockayne patients, at a young age, experience things we can see in elderly people, such as Parkinson's and Alzheimer's. People are interested in this, and it can help with funding."

Dr Theil's research into DNA repair disorders is utterly brilliant, and he does a fantastic job of demonstrating to the world that our children's problems are everyone's problems. Fixing them is a priority, and it should be a priority for everyone. He says that our children 'teach us how normal aging works'. And he's bang on the money.

There are teaching moments constantly to be had at Amy and Friends. I'm sure every parent of a child with Cockayne Syndrome will tell you how much they've learnt from their child. I think it's clear in this book how much I learnt from Amy. I learnt to be stronger, I learnt to be compassionate, and I learnt to appreciate the small things.

Dr Theil also credits Amy and Friends when it comes to needing information quickly. If he notices something significant in his lab, he can contact all of the families in Amy and Friends to see if they have experienced the same issue. We are all too willing to help him in any way we can.

On top of this, he talks beautifully about our precious kids:

"Meeting these children definitely changed my life in the sense that I became much more caring, much more social, and empathetic."

He also calls out my wonderful husband, noting correctly that, 'Mark has also had a huge impact.'

It's true!

He has!

He has!

When asked to describe Amy, he says:

"She was a bit naughty. She made a lot of jokes, and I like that personally. She was very much into interacting with all of the other families. She came to the Netherlands, and if there was a performance put on for them, she'd interact with them and make naughty jokes, and everyone laughed because she was really funny."

I know what he's thinking of here. He's thinking of a little show that was put on for us that was a bit, well, the level wasn't quite right. To put it bluntly, they were singing nursery rhymes to people with Cockayne who'd rather be watching Coronation Street. So when they gave everyone tea cups, sang Tea For Two, and pretended to pour tea out of a teapot into each person's cup, Amy wasn't having it. You know how much Amy likes tea. When no tea got poured into her cup, she looked over at me and shouted, 'WHAT THE **** IS THIS?' And Dr Theil creased up.

Dr Theil and I attend 'speed dating with pharmaceutical companies', kindly organised by Aspire Bioscience whose founder, Ron Jortner never gives up helping us, he says, 'he loves complicated and boy are we complicated!' Dr Theil and I often get put on what I refer to as The Naughty Table, and it's exactly where we belong.

He also offers hope and clarity to parents who have had none from their doctors. He offers to look into cases that have been neglected or abandoned. And when parents cry from feeling overwhelmingly grateful, he wraps them in a bear hug.

Our conferences also played a big part in setting up our London clinic. Dr Shehla Mohammed attends them diligently, and the families adore her. She's wonderful with them. She has, after all, dedicated her life to extremely vulnerable children with complex medical needs. She was the head of both the clinic and the laboratories where she worked, but she has always found the time to come to our conferences. She has over 30 years of experience working with children with extraordinarily rare genetic conditions, yet she has never stopped listening and valuing what patients and their families have to say. Here she is talking about our conferences in an informal chat:

"I was going to Amy and Friends conferences, getting suggestions and some really helpful pointers from parents. We told them we were designing this clinic, what would they like to see there?"

And she listened! And implemented! And built our clinic from the ground up. A clinic that functions at the top level, not just for the families with Cockayne, but for the clinicians too. It's a monumental feat!

CHAPTER 15: THE SCIENTISTS

Let's get specific now. I'm going to tell you a little bit about our latest conference, our 19th. It was unfortunately monsoon season in Blackpool at that time, but the inside of The Village Hotel was nicely climate-controlled. Aside however, from Professor Lehmann's room, which was too cold the first night and then uncomfortably hot the second after they fixed his thermostat. After lunch on the Friday, Mark gathers all of the scientists into a conference room. Many of them give talks on their latest research, and others are encouraged to weigh in. It's phenomenal.

If you've ever heard an outstanding neurologist present his research, then open it up for a discussion that's led by an award-winning geneticist with a brilliant nutritionist backing him up, then you'll know just how dynamic multidisciplinary discussions can be, especially when we are dealing with some of the finest minds in the world.

It's extremely unusual to have a meeting with so many great minds from different fields. One scientist pointed out that when you go to conferences for mainstream diseases such as Alzheimer's, there are often hundreds of scientists all from the same discipline, and the ability to have meaningful discussion is hindered. By having cherry-picked clinicians from different fields all get together, things really get moving.

So, what did they discuss this year?

Well, Mark chaired it, as usual. He opened up with a short talk about Amy and Friends and what he expected from the conference, which was Transparency, Collaboration, Sensitivity, Input, and Integrity. To be honest, all of the scientists there are also exemplary human beings with a moral compass so correct that it points directly to wherever Dolly Parton happens to be standing. Dolly's brilliant, isn't she? So, in sum, they were all happy with Mark's opening decree.

Then the talks began.

Dr Mohammed started off with our clinic's history, amongst other things. She mentioned our most recent move towards Bloom Syndrome, another DNA repair disorder like Cockayne and TTD. Bloom also inhibits growth and causes sun-sensitivity, but comes with the addition of cancer in the early years.

She talked about recent trends for rare diseases being named after the error in the underlying gene that is affected rather than after the person who discovered it. Dr Cockayne in particular has a name that has unfortunate associations.

The condition is named after Professor Alfred Cockayne, a paediatrician who worked at Great Ormond Street Hospital for Children, who first described the association of a particular group of symptoms affecting a number of body systems in 1946.

She also showed a map of Cockayne Syndrome cases in the UK. It turns out that Cockayne appears in clusters in certain areas. The patients are ethnically diverse, and most of the clusters surround teaching hospitals.

Is this suggestive that there may be more people with Cockayne that are undiagnosed? The team in London is working actively to ensure there is awareness of the condition and equity of access to the specialist clinic if families wish to be seen by clinicians with knowledge and experience of looking after children with Cockayne Syndrome.

And you'd be amazed how many times parents come to me for a diagnosis, because their doctors are not open to the possibility of it, just as my doctors weren't open to it thirty flipping years ago. So, anyone reading this, thinking things have changed since Amy was a kid, will be disappointed.

Some of them haven't changed.

I've lost count of the number of parents that have come to me with their children that I've sent off to their GPs with the message, 'Tell your doctor that Jayne says it's Cockayne.'

So far, it's worked. It's been the kick up the backside they've needed to send off for the tests.

Let's move on to Dr Abiona. Dr Abiona brings his guitar everywhere and sings like someone has coated his vocal chords in honey and pictures of Barry White. He stood to talk about tremors in children with Cockayne and his research into the best ways to mitigate them. He made the interesting point that often parents don't know their child has tremors. This is sometimes because tremors can often be interpreted as their child's natural movements. They can also be tricky to spot because most of the time it's most noticeable when eating with a knife and fork. This is when Amy's tremors were at their most obvious and distressing. However, once you take into account that many children with Cockayne are tube-fed, suddenly that chance to notice a tremor disappears. He talked sympathetically about the side effects of medications for tremors and highlighted that the quality of the children's lives was paramount.

Our occupational therapist, Dr Strudwick spoke up to say that there needs to be an improved standardised measure for tremors. Professor Hoeijmakers noted that tremors in his lab mice stop when the amount of calories they consume are significantly dropped. This was confirmed by our nutritionist, Julia Hopkins, who has also noted its impact.

As Julia reminded us all, it is a fine balance between getting the right amount of nutrition and calories, and this will need to be developed on an individual basis for each child, depending on how Cockayne Syndrome is affecting them.

Professor Kang talked about the usefulness of MRI scans of children with Cockayne. He wants to expand his data set to further his research and asked for clinicians to help by sharing MRI scans or by obtaining MRIs of their patients when it is feasible and clinically appropriate, as an MRI usually requires sedation or general anaesthesia in patients with Cockayne Syndrome.

Dr Van Ierland spoke about her clinic in Rotterdam, our sister clinic. She discussed setting it up but then displayed images of patients she had with unusual symptoms, one of which was an X-ray showing sclerotic bone lesions. She asked if anyone had encountered them before. The room came alive with advice from clinicians who had seen something similar. And owing to Mark, his presence as a father of a child with Cockayne, his insistence on sensitivity, and the scientists' kind natures, those children's medical issues were dealt with empathy, hope, and great care.

Dr Higgs talked about his work at Birmingham University and ended with an offer to let any interested scientists use their facilities to further their research.

Professor Ogi and Dr Theil discussed their research and ideas on how defects in DNA repair lead to Cockayne Syndrome. They came at it from two different angles, and watching these great minds declare war on Cockayne was enough to give you goosepimples.

Dr Le May showed his genetic research into a more accurate diagnosis of Cockayne. This will allow parents and carers to know which type of Cockayne their child or loved one has and serve to predict the future of their disorder.

And diagnosis, more accurate diagnosis is so important. Think back to the mother who had her baby taken away from her. Diagnosis would have stopped that. Despite that incident, things are improving all the time, and these scientists are the reason why. Dr Mohammed mentioned an apparent emerging trend utilising current technology, which is facilitating earlier diagnosis.

Dr Le May talked to me about making constant small steps forward, and he's right. A child was recently diagnosed at just four months old, and it's the earliest diagnosis so far. So, I'd say those small steps are, in terms of science and in terms of parents, HUGE.

Dr Le May loves our conferences. He says that our scientists are collaborative, not competitive, and that it's a big achievement for Amy and Friends. Plus, he admires our children and their families, calling them brave and resilient. Whenever he comes to our conferences and watches our children dancing, playing, bashing each other with balloon animals while collapsing into giggles, it reminds him exactly why he's here, exactly why he does what he does, and it only motivates him even harder. He loves our kids, and the feeling is mutual, Dr Le May! Your optimism and hard work are infectious!

So after all of these great scientists talk, it's Mark's tiny little job to work out how to translate it all into layman's terms to tell the families of the children and loved ones with Cockayne. The hall is always packed for this bit. Our brilliant carers take the kids out on an adventure. Shout out to Mr B, who is excellent with the kids. Former cop, former PE teacher, current absolute marshmallow of a man, because he's soft as anything with our children and can win any kid over.

Right, packed hall, Mark up front summing up all of the scientists' discussions, which fill everyone with such hope. I'm not talking about unrealistic hope, the sort you read about in the newspapers 'BLUEBERRIES HALT ALZHEIMER'S IN ITS TRACKS!' for example. I'm talking about the sort of hope you get from witnessing science move forward, like Dr Le May's small steps. The sort of hope that comes from seeing such great minds work so hard for our kids.

It's incredible.

We don't know when a cure will come, but Professor Lehmann, a man who says it's impossible to put a date on it, does marvel at how far they have come since 1980:

"If you'd actually told me, in 1980 what we can do now, I'd have said you're on a different planet, there's no way, you're in cloud cuckoo land."

And that in itself is just so damn hopeful. Remember when I was told it was Amy Syndrome? Look how different things are!

Then, it's time for parents and carers to ask questions.

We had one family from Australia, who really stood out. They've really been struggling to get enough care for their gorgeous little boy, and had travelled all of this way to meet other families and get help from our scientists. They had one question in particular for Dr Harrison.

I've not mentioned Dr Harrison yet, so I'll take the opportunity now. He's our specialist children's dentist. He looks after all of our kids' teeth at our clinic, and it's a seriously impressive feat. Amy hated the dentist. I mean, really hated it. She hated being interrupted while watching Coronation Street, too, but her hatred of dentists was on a whole different level. Her dental appointments were always painful and unpleasant. So at her first meeting with Dr Harrison, I told him, 'She won't open her mouth.'

I was wrong.

I'll admit now that I was wrong because Dr Harrison got her to open her mouth in no time. One trick he uses is to hand little mirrors out to the kids and ask them to use them to look at their own teeth. Before you know it, they're opening their mouths so wide that Dr Harrison can see all the way back to their breakfast.

So, what was his response to this lovely Australian mother who told him that her son hated dentists so much he bit the dentist's little mirror off its little stick and choked on it?

Well, he was fab. He talked about dentists of children with Cockayne needing to be more open to the idea of using sedation to help them through complicated dental work. He also spoke about other issues, such as weakness in the muscles around the mouth, which was exactly what I was talking about in Chapter 3, and how it impacts babies' ability to latch on and feed.

The dental implications of this can mean that teeth grow outwards. He applauded the orthodontist who thought outside the box and was willing to give braces to their son, but lamented that the correction may not be permanent.

Every audience member sympathised. Dental issues are rampant in our community, and finding an understanding dentist is hard, not least when your child ages out of children's special care and has to wait for an adult specialist dentist. So three cheers for Dr Harrison, he makes a big difference in our clinic with his little mirrors.

When this Australian family asked how they could receive more help for their son back home, they were given the details of a geneticist with knowledge of Cockayne to contact down under. Perfect! Dr Mohammed also took this opportunity to talk about how they are working on writing more leaflets with guidelines for Cockayne for clinicians to access all around the world.

They also spoke about attending more and more paediatric conferences, spreading the word of Cockayne, which is what I'm doing in my own way right now! It's brilliant news. I only hope they include our epic wheelchair races at the clinic while they're at it.

The questions came thick and fast, and every clinician had something to say. Kudos to Phillipa Sellar, our clinic's wonderful specialist nurse, for carefully giving a detailed answer to a family whose teenage son was starting to struggle with hormones.

The fear of cancer was raised, and how parents can possibly know if their child is developing it. Professor Kang used this moment to highlight the importance of data collection to better help predict and diagnose cancer in its early stages in children who cannot tell you if something has started to not quite feel right. This is where he talked about the importance of listening to parents, and he's right! He's right! If something has changed, if something is different in our children, we, the parents and the carers, are the only ones who can spot it.

When your child has such a complicated myriad of medical issues, you are the ones who know what your child's 'normal' is. Remember Amy's increased appetite? The changes might not seem particularly important, you might simply be talking sausages, but they're vital to report.

Our nurse, Phillipa spoke insightfully about this both at the conference and to me in an informal chat. Here she talks about nurses' roles in recognising the unique wellness of their patients:

"Nurses provide continuity. I know people can't help it when registrars change every year. People change jobs. You see somebody different even in a GP practice now, and that can be really difficult for families when they're trying to demonstrate the complexity of their child's condition. So by offering continuity and consistency, we can build rapport, build relationships, and build a level of trust. We know from research that it actually improves outcomes for our patients because people begin to share more with you if they have a relational component with the clinician. They'll share things that are smaller and not wait until they're bigger problems, which is how you prevent hospital admissions. We build the ability of the team around patients to know what their unique wellness is, especially if they can't articulate it for themselves."

Finally, Dr Mohammed dealt with the most sensitive question of all. The one that plagues every one of us.

'How long will my child live?'

It's a question filled with desperation and fear. It's one Dr Mohammed dealt with gently. She told them, she told the whole room that it's variable, that it's constantly changing due to science and medicine moving forward. That it is not a set thing, not any longer. Then she told that particular parent that she would speak to them after to get a better understanding of their child and so a better idea of their life expectancy.

You could have heard a pin drop.

It was an emotional moment for the families.

And so we concluded it all with a funny moment and a ridiculous sing-along, and woosh up goes the energy in the room again.

As scientists and families walked out of the hall, people stopped to ask more personal questions, and our lovely scientists answered them all, with no hurry, just with sympathy and respect.

The children came back ten minutes later, and that's when the party started!

This year, we had the fancy dress theme of music through the ages, and nobody disappointed. There were at least four Freddie Mercurys of varying ages. Several Michael Jacksons. A stunning

KISS group costume, featuring my brilliant Laura, who was there fresh after castrating a Boxer dog, and of course, my boys and their mates dressed as the Spice Girls. My favourite costume of the night was one of our little boys dressed in white, with feathers and diamonds, and crystal-studded glasses, being Elton John. His wheelchair had been turned into a white grand piano, so he looked like he was performing wherever he went. Genius!

There was dancing, there was singing, from Billy Hui's fantastic choir, the one Amy loved so much, from an Elvis impersonator, and from Dr Abiona, Soji, who performed, amongst others, a song he had composed specially for the event. Want to see a mum in fancy dress twerking before one of the world's most eminent scientists? Come along! Want to see a dance off between two of our volunteers that was taken so very competitively that the worm was performed on the dancefloor? Come along! Where else could you see this!

It was ridiculous, it was hilarious, and the karaoke afterward was damn good fun. At any moment, you could be the lucky receiver of a hug from parents and children alike. And when one of our kids climbs into your lap and wraps your arms around them, I'm telling you now, you won't want to let go.

We are absolutely a family. We hand out a brochure with photos and names for everyone who attends. Our volunteers who come time after time and our families and scientists. Aleisha, one of Amy's dear friends who lived with us for a while was there, making our children laugh, making our parents laugh. She is a treasure.

Ami Knowles was there too, with her adorable, little, energetic whirlwind of a daughter. She also lived with us for a while and was one of Amy's close friends. She has this to say about clinicians:

"They won't find a cure if they don't work together with the families. It's got to be a joint effort."

Professor Kang agrees. Dr Abiona agrees. Dr Mohammed agrees. Dr Theil and Dr Le May agree. All of our scientists agree! So you should listen to her.

Our conferences are a bit like visiting a magical land, where you can talk to anyone, where your smile is always returned. Where, if you break down for a moment, you get hugs from every direction. It really hits home when it finishes and you head to Tesco and beam at everyone you pass only to be looked at like you're a weirdo.

Let's hear from Dr Abiona. Dr Abiona is brilliant at our clinic. Talking to some doctors can feel a bit like a boxing match. Talking to Dr She's-faking-her-leg-dragging-due-to-poor-self-image felt more like a shark attack. But Dr Abiona? Talking to Dr Abiona feels like a warm hug. This is what he had to say about joining Amy and Friends:

"When I first got wind of Amy and Friends, I was a little shell-shocked because I wasn't used to the positivity. I mean, I knew that within Cockayne Syndrome one part of the features of the children can be that they're very happy. They can be quite jovial. But I didn't realise that that was going to translate to their parents as well.'

What a great point. He's right. We all take our cue from our kids. They're happy kids and they want to have fun, and so we, as parents, well, we want that too.

If you want to be a part of this, take a look here: https://www.facebook.com/amyandfriendsCockayneSyndromeandTTD

Of course there are sad moments.

We never forget our kids who have passed away. We have a memorial wall full of their pictures. When Jade got up and sang 'Run' by Snow Patrol, we all stood, holding a photo of a dear child who we've lost. Nothing hits like it. Nothing hits like holding the picture of a beautiful, smiling little face as high as you can, telling the world that you are not going to let them go.

None of us is going to let them go.

We will remember them all forever.

It's our little moment to cry. And we do. We all do. It is a sadness that you need to see to understand. If you have seen, if you have seen a man break down on the ground crying for his beloved sons, if you have heard a woman's voice, filled with pain, call out, 'My son. My son.' before being piled on with hugs. Then you'll have an idea of the pain and the strength of our families.

If you even got a glimpse of it, when they come in future to your hospital, you would never let anyone treat them like shit again.

Even our karaoke can break your heart. I'm telling you now, you've never heard anything sang right until you've heard it sung slightly out of tune, with enthusiasm, by a child who will never reach adulthood.

One particular jump from fun to sadness came from a little boy and his dad. His dad had raised a whopping amount of money for Amy and Friends after his son challenged him, a man who hates jogging, to run 60 half marathons in 60 days. When brought up on stage to raucous applause, his son opened his mouth to issue another challenge. I'm not entirely sure what it was going to be. It started with 'Run a hundred–' before his dad clamped his hands firmly over his gob to shut him up. Those two are hilarious. That boy looks at his dad like he's his hero, and is totally unaware that his dad is looking back at him the same way.

They caused some of the loudest laughs of the weekend.

But after Jade sang 'Run', he turned and matter-of-factly said, 'One day you'll hold my photo up.'

It destroyed everyone in earshot.

All of this, all of this you need to know. Because it will make you kinder to the people who come to your clinic, and, if you're kinder, you'll work harder to help.

Once you experience it, you'll want to run 60 half marathons in 60 days to find a cure.

It'll make you want to jump out of aeroplanes. It'll make you want to climb bloody Everest. Every scientist in the building would scale Everest without hesitation. Every parent, every sibling, every innocent bystander who accidentally crashes the party because they've been kicked out of the pub. We'd all climb Everest.

In fact, Everest is nothing compared to Cockayne.

If only finding a cure could be so easy. We'd all have sherpas on speed dial.

Just in case any of this makes you want to do a fundraiser of any sort, here's where you can get the information you need:

https://amyandfriends.org/digital-fundraising-pack/

CHAPTER 16: COCKAYNE SYNDROME AS AN ADULT

Let's jump back into Amy's life. By this point, Amy was an adult. For clinicians trying to help people with Cockayne Syndrome, it was a bit like unknown territory. So many patients with Cockayne tragically pass away before they reach ten years old. So doctors found themselves dealing with a disorder they may have been hearing about for the first time, with a patient who had reached adulthood against the odds.

It was like unknown territory squared.

And two things made Amy's life a lot harder.

1. She was having to deal with more debilitating symptoms than ever.
2. The NHS didn't have any way to cater to her.

This chapter will deal with one particularly inept moment, but mainly it's going to look at how the care of the NHS breaks down when dealing with an adult who is the size of a young child.

This is a problem with the system and was no doubt frustrating for the clinicians involved, too.

Let's start with taking blood.

Regular blood tests were something Amy underwent constantly. It's unfortunately a common part of having Cockayne Syndrome.

Let's talk, however, about one particular blood test Amy had been sent to the phlebotomy for. It was a test of her glucose levels to see how well we were handling her diabetes.

The girl on the desk was chewing gum and had a bottle of Coke that appeared to be glued to her left hand. She pulled up Amy's details on her computer and pointed to the plastic seating.

Amy and I were in the sort of place where it seemed we spent most of our time. A hospital waiting room.

I spy with my little eye, something beginning with P.

It's piles again isn't it.

This time, Amy wasn't just bored, she was terrified.

When I say that, I don't say it lightly.

Amy was flat out, hands down, the bravest person I have ever met. But she was terrified of blood tests.

She wasn't scared because she had a phobia. She wasn't squeamish about needles. She was scared because blood tests hurt her. They bloody hurt her! She was now an adult, attending the adult phlebotomy department, so they used adult-sized needles on her.

However, Amy was the size of a seven-year-old. So the needles were too big.

This wasn't just absolutely awful for Amy, it was really blinking difficult for the clinicians. They never hit a vein first time. It would take try after try after try.

I shall never forget one particularly difficult appointment where the phlebotomist failed eight times to find the vein in one arm, and started in on Amy's other arm instead.

Amy leapt off the bed, ran across the room, and hid in the cupboard!

This was probably a first for the phlebotomy department.

Blood tests are rotten. Nobody likes having them done. Most phlebotomists know this and are lovely. The brilliant ones are so superb at distracting conversation that they were probably hairdressers in a past life.

'Clench your fist for me. Been anywhere nice on your holidays?'

Perfect.

But when your equipment isn't suitable for the patient, as it wasn't for Amy, no amount of talking about Magaluf is going to cut it.

It might seem small in the long run of things.

In fact, I imagine it appears extremely small in the face of Parkinson's, tumours, seizures, hearing and sight loss, and all the rest of Pandora's Box of Cockayne Syndrome complications. However, to our kids, blood tests are a big thing. They're a big thing to fear, because they're going to be difficult and painful, and most of our kids really dread them. They wake up in the morning with the sort of butterflies you have before a maths test. The sort of nerves you feel when you've got your driving test. Or that dull aching panic you have when you get to the airport and start to wonder if you've left the hob on.

We deal with this in our clinic in a way that has proved to be more successful than we had even hoped.

We take bloods from all the children first thing in the morning. This means we have the results before they go home in the evening. We learnt to do it like this the hard way, when one child's blood tests came back critical while they were already on the train and halfway home.

We didn't do that again!

So, all bloods are taken first thing.

We always use butterfly needles. Even our few adult patients are small. Butterfly needles are best; they mean a significant reduction in pain and an easier job getting them in a vein.

Finally, we have so many fun things for the kids to do after, arts, crafts, toys, the sort of shenanigans that sees eminent geneticist, Professor Lehmann, doing Superman gymnastics on the waiting room floor.

https://amyandfriends.org/professor-lehmann-superman/

Plus, there are biscuits.

Frankly, I have come to see it as the only way to take tea.

When the kids come to our clinic in London, they're so excited for all the fun they're going to have, they don't seem to mind the blood tests at the start. They're always looking forward to what's coming next, so they don't spend too long worrying about them.

I'm going to interrupt myself here to talk about a peculiarity of Cockayne Syndrome that has nothing to do with phlebotomy, because children with Cockayne don't just live life at a sort of rapid, fast-forward sort of pace; they're also always looking to the future. A kid with Cockayne Syndrome is always asking, 'What's next?'

They could be having a great time, but they'll still want to know what's happening next. Amy was absolutely like this. She'd be only a few sips into a cup of tea before she was enquiring into the possibility of the next brew.

It's just a funny little quirk of Cockayne.

At our Amy and Friends' conferences, we understand that no matter how jampacked with activities and fun the day is, the kids will always be asking, 'What's next?' So, we make sure we have a clear itinerary in order for every parent and child to be able to see exactly what's next!

Right, where were we? Blood tests! If you're dealing with a patient with Cockayne Syndrome and you have to take blood, know that there's a chance they're going to be terrified due to nasty past experiences, potentially with needles that were the wrong size. Use a butterfly needle, if you can get your mitts on one. It'll make a huge difference to your ability to get the vein and to their pain levels.

Don't expect them to run away and hide in your cupboard, though! Our Amy always had a different way of going about things.

So, back to us, in that waiting room, waiting for a blood test. We'd just come from a check-up with a doctor for her diabetes, who was great. He'd referred us over for the blood test, and that's how we found ourselves checking in with the girl with her gum and her Coke.

She reads Amy's file, spots Cockayne Syndrome, and gets hung up on it. She tells us she doesn't know what colour bottle to put the Cockayne blood into.

I tell her that Amy has diabetes. That we're here for a blood sugar test. She's just checking her blood sugar, so she can use the bottle for that.

She tells me, like I'm a bit dim, 'Yeah, but it says she's got Cockayne Syndrome.' And she immediately starts phoning around trying to find out which vial they use for Cockayne Syndrome.

Now, if someone with diabetes also had cancer, and came in to check their blood sugar, I'm pretty sure they'd put it into the vials for blood sugar, not a vial that is specifically for Non-Hodgkin's Lymphoma, who needs their blood sugar testing.

Cockayne Syndrome just sends people into a panic. We sat for over an hour and a half, watching her chew gum and drink Coke while she waited to hear which vial should be used for Amy's blood sugar test.

In the end, I turned to Amy and suggested we head out for a cuppa instead of continuing to wait in that drab room.

I called the lovely doctor who'd referred us to phlebotomy on the way to the café. His secretary answered. I told her exactly what had happened and that we were off to get a cup of tea, and that we weren't going to come back for the blood test.

She said, 'I don't blame you.'

So, we went and got a cup of tea instead.

And a biscuit!

Right, what's next?

Ahh yes, The House of Commons!

CHAPTER 17: THE IDEA FOR A CLINIC

This is where Mark and I get to speak at the House of Commons. You see, Amy and Friends was going from strength to strength, but the NHS was in a constant state of chaos and panic when it came to caring for Amy and all of the other kids in our charity. Most of the clinicians we met were just doing their job, which isn't an easy thing, and we appreciated it. Some of them were phenomenal. But some were abusive (boos and hisses to that neurologist et al). However, good or bad, they were all hindered by a lack of communication and a lack of consistency. You know what it's like, you never see the same doctor twice. That's not a doctor problem, that's a system problem.

So the NHS was failing our kids.

It's not just blood test needles that were a problem for Cockayne patients who were adults whilst being the size of children. The adult department of hospitals just weren't set up for them, and it felt sometimes like we were slipping through gaps the NHS didn't even realise needed spackling.

I'm telling you, lino wallpaper. It should be a thing.

So when one of the wonderful men at The Docker's Club turned out to have an important connection, we found ourselves standing before The House of Commons on Rare Diseases Day, pleading our case. Mark talked about the scientific side of Cockayne. I spoke about the lived experience.

We needed help.

Serious help.

And we needed it now!

The place went silent. Nobody would look at me. Nobody wanted to even catch my eye, because nobody wanted to help.

It was excruciating.

I felt like this was my last hope. I had run out of ideas if this didn't work, I was going to have to go back to the drawing board.

And then.

In the midst of the silence and the lowered heads.

A woman stood up, took my hand, looked me in the eye, and said, 'I'll help you.'

Ladies, gentlemen, and non-binary readers, allow me to introduce again to you the extraordinary, the incomparable, the absolute genius who was the clinical lead in The Houses of Parliament that day, Dr Shehla Mohammed.

It was the moment that changed everything.

Spielberg couldn't have directed it better!

You're going to love Dr Mohammed, and you know you can trust me in this because I was right when I told you you were going to love Professor Kang, wasn't I?

Dr Shehla Mohammed, who wrote the foreword to this book, was and still is absolutely pivotal to the creation of our London Clinic. She's amazing.

I knew from our conferences that our children needed such a clinic. Bringing clinicians together from different disciplines is the best way to deal with such medically complex patients. So I knew it could work. What I didn't know at this point was how to go about setting it up. I was impatient to get it up and running. When your child has Cockayne Syndrome, you're painfully aware of how much time is passing. Unfortunately, in order to create a clinic that would be stable and lasting, it needed to be done right. And that took time.

I was lucky, I had two geneticist giants helping me, Dr Mohammed and Professor Lehmann. Plus, Dr Mohammed and Professor Lehmann, with other colleagues, already had a multidisciplinary clinic set up for children with Xeroderma Pigmentosum, (XP), so Dr Mohammed knew how well they worked and how to go about setting them up. It seemed like it would all fall into place easily.

But it would take far longer than I had ever anticipated.

Not only that, but I felt that with every passing hospital appointment, the need for a specialised clinic only became more stark.

Now, I have purposefully written this book in a way that you are hopefully finding entertaining, and up to this point, introduction aside, not made you too sad. Angry, perhaps, but not too distressed. This next bit is going to get sad, however it all ends well. The reason it gets upsetting is because Amy starts to lose her sight. This was extremely distressing all round, and I had to put a brave face on it.

My memories of this time were that I was desperate for her to remember how things looked, things most people take for granted, like colours.

I'd point out sunflowers and tell her, 'Look at how beautiful and yellow those sunflowers are. Try to remember it so when your sight goes and I describe something as yellow as a sunflower, you'll know exactly what I'm talking about.'

It was profoundly heartbreaking, but I learnt a lot from those moments. They taught me to take great joy in small things such as a sunflower by the side of the road. I began to appreciate my surroundings more.

Amy has taught me so much. How to be strong, how to be assertive, how to be compassionate, and how to enjoy the small things. Because the small things are the big things, aren't they?

All of my children have taught me so much. And while this book is about the life experience of people with Cockayne Syndrome, I need to tell you quickly that Amy's brothers and sister have also taught me so much. They have shown me what it looks like to be a carer from birth. They all took to it so naturally and have, as I said earlier, gone into caring professions. My journey with Cockayne Syndrome started when Amy was born, but for them, well they experienced it their entire lives. Their continuing help with Amy and Friends is selfless and wonderful, because it's not easy, not when the children are so very sick or when they're nearing the end of their lives. And nobody would blame them if they decided they'd had a skinful of Cockayne, if they were done with it. As Amy's health worsened and the number of hospital appointments increased, we were, at times, almost like two families. Me looking after Amy, them with their dad Mark out doing fun things. That cannot have been easy for them. In fact, it was extremely hard for all of us. So, if they decided that they wanted to live fun, frivolous lives, travelling or partying, not having any responsibilities, doing whatever they wanted, it'd be understandable, wouldn't it? Instead, they all have chosen to help and to care for others, and I don't think there can be a more noble way of living life than that. So while this book is about Amy and how Cockayne Syndrome impacted her life and mine, never forget that there is a whole family behind this book who are absolutely amazing.

Back to it, Amy's eyesight was deteriorating fast, and it was due to salt and peppering of the retina.

Awful. Unfair. But glasses can help, right?

Well, yes, if you're an adult with the issue it's easy to get them fixed. But when you're an adult that's the size of a seven-year-old, the NHS cannot help you. You can't stay in the kids' wards. You can't be seen by the kids' doctors. However, they also can't use the equipment for adults on you, because it's way too big.

The NHS ophthalmologist Amy saw was absolutely lovely. He was brilliant. And despite the fact that he really wanted to help, when he informed us he couldn't due to their equipment not being suitable for her, Amy turned to me and said:

"The NHS doesn't exist for us."

And despite the hundreds of appointments we had had throughout her life, she was right really, wasn't she?

Watching, helpless, as your daughter loses her sight was horrific, but here's where things get better. We met an excellent ophthalmologist, another one of those streetlights shining in what was literally fog, in terms of Amy's eyesight. He worked for Specsavers, and he had child-appropriate equipment that he had no hesitation in using for our adult Amy.

He prescribed baby sized thick glasses for her eyes, and she could see again.

Shall we hallelujah again?

For Amy, for Leonard Cohen, and Billy Hui's choir.

I think we should.

Halle-bloody-lujah!

The clinic that we set up in London has a great ophthalmologist, handpicked by Dr Mohammed, who takes care of all of our patients' optical needs. They're used to all the problems Cockayne Syndrome throws up, and they have the right-sized equipment to deal with it.

I may at times sound like I'm angry at the NHS when they can't cater to people with Cockayne Syndrome. I know I come across like

I am furious when I talk about people like Dr ****head, and the neurologist that threw the paper on the ground, and the awful paediatrician who force-fed baby Amy like he was going to use her for foie gras.

And I am.

I am angry.

But there were many brilliant clinicians too. Shout out to the kidney specialist at Alder Hay in their Urology Department. Amy had had high blood pressure since the age of 13, she was put on blood pressure medication but nobody had taken any tests to work out why it was so high. With the medication her blood pressure was under control, but the moment she stopped taking it, it'd go through the roof again. Well, not through my roof, she'd have to get through an attic full of boxes that I haven't unpacked since we moved here, but through someone's roof who has a nice, clear attic.

This superb specialist finally scanned her kidneys and found that one kidney was only working at two-thirds of its capacity. The other kidney was tiny and not working properly either. On discovering this, the specialist told us he was going to take over her care completely because she needed to be taking a different medication on account of her kidneys leaking protein. That medication really helped make her feel so much better. His care was top-notch, and it absolutely led to her life being prolonged that little bit longer.

Only a little.

But the small things are everything.

A few years later, we met a girl with Cockayne that also had kidney issues and so we told her to go to him. That family told us, after their appointment, that he had told them he had treated another girl with Cockayne Syndrome. Our Amy. And when they told him that she had passed away he cried. Just flat-out sobbed during their appointment. He is such a caring and clever man.

So, yes, there were many superb clinicians. And significantly, there were plenty of average doctors who were just trying to do their jobs and go home at the end of the day, which is perfectly reasonable! However, the way the NHS is set up hindered people who were actively trying to help.

I think the NHS is amazing.

I think it is struggling.

And I'm afraid, I think in Amy's words, there are just times when the NHS doesn't exist for a specific type of patient. Unfortunately, people with Cockayne Syndrome frequently fall into that category.

So, when I say 'In our clinics we have fixed this problem', I don't say this in the way one might say, 'Ner ner ner ner nerrr.' I'm saying, we opened a clinic to help the NHS with patients with Cockayne Syndrome. We take a burden to the tune of four million pounds off the NHS. We collate all the information, and we make it easier for doctors all over the country to know what they're doing when it comes to patients with Cockayne.

One particular thing we do at our clinic that makes the lives of hardworking NHS clinicians easier is the creation of an illness passport. Every child we see gets a laminated outline of their illness. This can then be presented to doctors in appointments and tells them quickly and accurately everything about that patient. We update their passports to keep them accurate, and they've been a real game-changer. Cockayne causes such a myriad of issues, right across the board, that having the information presented in a passport saves time and stops any kind of confusion.

Shehla describes it like this:

"Paula Sullivan and Phillipa Sellar worked with parents and the clinical team to develop a care passport. It's a comprehensive record of the child's medical needs on a day-to-day basis. It contains what precautions may need to be taken when they're in hospital. It's a complete passport, which means that they don't have to recite the story yet again to someone who is unfamiliar with the condition."

Phillipa Sellar takes a look at the impact our passport makes on the other side of the table:

"On the whole, the feedback that we get from people like registrars, who are in A&E at 3 o'clock in the morning on a Sunday, when they're presented with a child with a syndrome they've never heard of, is overwhelmingly positive. They're really pleased to get some support and help in the form of a document. That's not to malign the great work and representation parents and carers can give. They're experts in their child's needs. But somehow, in the stress of being in the middle of A&E, having to relay the child's information numerous times, it's extremely helpful to have something tangible to hand over to clinicians."

So you see, we help the NHS, and we make the work the clinicians within it do, easier.

I don't dislike them at all.

They are the reason Amy lived for so long.

We have met many utterly wonderful people in the NHS, and as I have Open Access to all hospitals that are caring for patients with Cockayne, I personally work with them all the time. Within the NHS are thousands of people, working hard, with altruism and compassion. We aim to demystify Cockayne for them, which is best for both doctor and patient.

To continue to hammer home how much we needed this clinic, let's take a look at another example of Cockayne sufferers' needs not being met by the NHS. Incontinence. It is a bloody awful aspect of Cockayne Syndrome. It's not fair, and the impact it has on their dignity is distressing. But after a certain length of time, Cockayne Syndrome will start to affect the bladder and the bowels.

Life is already hard enough for them. This is a terrible thing for our patients to have to suffer. However, the NHS cannot provide our patients with any kind of incontinence pants or sheets.

When Amy was 22, she was the size, as I've previously stated, of a seven-year-old. The NHS refused to send us incontinence pull-up pants because they said even their smallest size would be too small. I asked, begged really, if they could please send us one to try. They insisted that they wouldn't fit her and refused to just send one out for us to check because the system only allowed her to send 200 at a time. If they ended up not fitting, they had no returns system for us to post them back.

So pull-up incontinence pants were a no-no.

But making a bright, intelligent, kind, and bursting with sass 22-year-old woman wear a nappy, laying her on her back and having to change her as if she were a baby was a wretched indignity that she and nobody deserves.

Okay, maybe some people deserve it.

Like Hitler, and Pol Pot, and Dr Throw-the-paper-on-the-floor.

If Hell exists, I'll know where to forward his mail.

The NHS also wouldn't send incontinence sheets out to Cockayne sufferers, and it would have saved many families from such distressing and economically difficult situations. Before our clinic opened, Amy and Friends helped families buy new bedding when the old stuff was so covered in faeces, the bin was the only place for them.

Sometimes clinicians focus on the big picture, the major organs, when the day-to-day hell of incontinence has a massive impact on the quality of life of not just the patient, but their carers too.

For some children with Cockayne Syndrome, incontinence hits them early, and we have one young boy who is in a mainstream school who struggles with it.

The NHS wouldn't provide him with pull-ups. Their reasoning was that he can and does go to the bathroom without issue. His problem was not that he was incapable of using a bathroom, his problem was that he couldn't always make it. They told him to go to the bathroom more often to avoid accidents.

That's not very helpful, is it?

It's not like this kid wanted to wet himself every day in front of his peers.

Their lives are hard enough. A pull-up that fits should not be too much to ask for.

Our clinic makes contact with local teams to ensure incontinence needs are met with dignity.

CHAPTER 18: CONSENT

This chapter is going to talk about a really difficult and constantly discussed issue.

Consent.

I'm sure you're all aware of how important consent is when it comes to doctors treating patients. It seems obvious to most of us that there must be consent before you even touch a patient, but it's not always the case. There are also some extremely grey areas where doctors will feel they have done what's right, while patients are left feeling violated.

Let's start by going back briefly to my C-section. I gave them consent to experiment on me, but it wasn't informed consent. I hadn't been fully briefed about how badly it could go. I also wasn't anywhere near the right headspace. I was at once elated that the last ultrasound had been normal, whilst terrified for my baby's survival at such an early stage. I had an extremely at-risk pregnancy, and everything was moving so fast that it was hard to take in anything they were saying.

So, in terms of consent, that was an extremely grey area. Feel free to discuss amongst yourselves what your opinion is of it. I don't have any real, lasting resentment of those doctors, but if they'd told me how horrific it was going to be, I'd have said, 'Hell no!'

Next, let's talk about consent done right. On one of our visits to Boston Children's Hospital, Amy's tremors had increased and were just awful. They started to fear that it wasn't something like Parkinson's. They were worried it was Huntington's. I'm not sure about you, but Huntington's is a word that never ceases to instil absolute dread in the pit of my stomach. The doctor at the hospital asked if they could do a lumbar puncture to find out if their fears were founded.

All of this was discussed with both Amy and me with great respect. Amy was around 15 at the time, and at no point did we feel any pressure to agree to it. I carefully asked him, 'If she has this lumbar puncture and it reveals that she does have Huntington's, can you help her?'

The doctor answered honestly with, 'No, but at least we'll know what she has.'

So I spoke to Amy. I told her that lumbar punctures could be awful procedures. That she could be in terrible pain after, and that the headaches can be horrific. All of this would be done just to get an answer to the Huntington's question. It wouldn't get her any help, just an answer.

The doctor sat patiently while we discussed it until Amy asked him a question that was so ridiculously typical of her.

She asked, 'Will it help other children if I have it done?'

He told her, 'Along the way, Amy, yes, it will help others.'

So she said, 'Do it.'

No hesitation.

When it came to helping other people, she never hesitated.

I even double checked with her, 'You're going to be in pain and it's not going to help you.'

But she stuck to her guns, 'It's okay. Do it.'

She was in such pain afterward. She was absolutely floored by it, but she looked up at me with the most beautiful smile and said, 'It's okay, Mum. I'm okay.'

I dare say that's consent done well. She knew it was going to be rough. She knew exactly why it was being done. And she was willing and able to go through with it.

Allow me to introduce to you consent example number three.

Amy was in a physiotherapy appointment with a physio we'd not met before. Amy is lying on the examination bed. She was physically quite weak at this stage of her life, but still strong in spirit. You'll be able to see this, because the physio did something that would immediately make most people freeze.

She climbed up onto the bed, straddled Amy, and started to manipulate her neck!

She didn't say a bloody word!

No warning of what she was about to do.

No asking consent.

Nothing!

She just leapt onto Amy.

I was horrified, but my mouth doesn't work as fast as Amy's, who immediately shouted at her, 'GET OFF ME YOU PERVE!'

That's my girl.

So, this case wasn't just a matter of consent done badly, it was a case of consent not asked for at all. This physiotherapist was a member of the NHS for crying out loud!

Let's move on to example four. It's at our clinic.

All of our specialist clinicians have been handpicked. They are all serious about gaining consent before touching a patient, and at times, they have to do tests that are unpleasant. I'd like to talk about one boy who came to us that needed a skin biopsy. He was scared, and with good reason. They're not very nice, are they?

Our clinician told him exactly what it would entail, with compassion. He talked kindly and gently, but he didn't sugarcoat it or make it seem like it was going to be nothing. Once consent was given, he carried out the biopsy with great care. I dare say all of our clinicians carry out their tests with love, and that makes all the difference. When nasty tests are done with such care, no patient feels violated.

Example five.

One of Amy's lovely friends was 26. Cockayne Syndrome had had a severe impact on her growth. She had the sweetest nature, was a dear friend, and she was the size of a two-year-old. When she started to seriously go into decline, she was taken to adult services and given CPR.

They utterly destroyed her body.

Breaking her bones as she died.

She had had an official, legally binding DNACPR/DNR in place.

Do Not Attempt Cardiopulmonary Resuscitation.

We know our children are going to pass away at some point. In Amy and Friends it is an awful, absolutely awful reality of Cockayne Syndrome that we see far too frequently. Not one parent is under the illusion that they won't. What we all want is the wish that I made when I tucked Amy into bed at 2 years old after being told she wouldn't live long.

Please don't let her suffer.

Amy's friend suffered horrifically. Far more than if she had simply passed from a Cockayne complication.

It was devastating.

Consent was nowhere to be seen.

Example six.

This one also includes a major way the NHS sometimes doesn't exist for people with Cockayne. It starts one evening when Amy started hiccupping and telling me that she didn't feel right. I gave her her prescribed acid reflux medicine, and she went to bed, but I couldn't settle. She didn't seem particularly ill, but something about her hiccups made me uncomfortable. I spent the night slipping in and out of her room, checking on her.

When she started making strange little noises of discomfort around 1 am, I ran into her room and she was sitting up in what can only be described as a scene from a horror movie. She had vomited black blood all over the walls, all over her bed, and all over herself and her hair.

She then informed me that she felt much better after that!

I was terrified, though! I called 999 and they took her to hospital with a suspected stomach bleed. So, they put an endoscope down her throat, with only a very mild sedative.

It was an adult-sized endoscope going down her child-sized throat, and it was horrific. Absolutely horrific. Her stomach, it turned out, was fine. Their hypothesis was that medication she'd taken at some point had irritated her stomach, causing a bleed, but it had subsequently healed, leaving the old blood behind.

Three weeks later it happened again. Black blood vomit everywhere. So, they told her they were going to repeat the endoscopy.

Amy freaked out. She told them, 'No.' She said she didn't want it. She was extremely distressed. I told them she had had an endoscopy last time and it hadn't shown anything, and that she didn't want it done again.

They didn't listen to her, an adult, who was refusing the procedure. They wouldn't listen to me, her mum, either.

Amy was beside herself with terror.

Finally, I told them I had Power of Attorney, just to get them to back down. But they were absolutely going to go ahead, without her or my consent, while she begged them not to do it.

And now we have our final example. Example number seven.

Amy's ultimate wish was to never be tube-fed. She had plenty of friends within Amy and Friends who were tube-fed, and she had a real horror of it.

She was 27 at this point.

She knew exactly what being tube-fed meant, and she couldn't bear the thought of it.

So, of course, as this chapter is all about consent, you've probably got the sinking realisation that she was going to end up living with one of her worst nightmares, against her will.

She said no to the feeding tube.

They overruled her.

They ignored her refusal.

They didn't bother getting consent.

They wheeled her into surgery and gave her a feeding tube.

And it was as bad as she feared. She was in agony with it. Abscesses developed all around it. It got to the point where an abscess would be burst every day in hospital so they could clean it and change the dressings.

If you have ever had an abscess, if you have ever known the horrific pain of an abscess, you'll understand how torturous it is. We couldn't even pick her up or hold her anymore because she was in too much pain.

She never complained.

She never damn complained.

They gave her that feeding tube without her consent, and she was never the same again. She was to pass away soon after, and it is so damn hard to even tell you about it. Cockayne Syndrome let her down, but there were so many times when clinicians made life harder for her.

Consent.

I know you would never touch a patient without it; but there are plenty of people out there that don't even think twice about it.

CHAPTER 19: THE CLINIC OPENS!

For years, Dr Shehla Mohammed, Professor Alan Lehmann, and I were working like mad to get the clinic up and running. I'm not sure I have ever doggedly pursued anything in my life the way I pursued that clinic. Every year we came closer to it, yet it still remained tantalisingly distant. Dr Mohammed took on the most. She is the one who knew how the system worked and how the funding application worked. I couldn't just get my dad to help me this time!

We became a decent team. She would call me into meetings so I could offer a peek into the lived experience of families with Cockayne Syndrome, Professor Lehmann provided scientific context. We edged forward bit by bit, drawing ever closer to the grant. In the meantime, I became adept at public speaking about Cockayne.

It turns out that when your child has a life-limiting disorder, you don't particularly get stressed about things like public speaking. Very few things make you panic. When someone comes to me freaking out about something, I ask two questions: 'Is anyone dying? Has anyone died?' And if the answer is no, then there's no need to panic. Once you surround yourself with children with Cockayne Syndrome, you realise that the everyday things are nothing to get worked up about. You find yourself not caring about stuff the rest of the world cares about. None of it matters. Holiday flights cancelled? Is it really a big deal? Your computer's deleted a week's worth of work? It doesn't really bother you when your child's kidneys start failing. All those adverts for perfume, and shampoo, and laundry detergent. I don't have time to sniff my blouse! I have hospital appointments to get to. It feels sometimes like we live in a different world to everyone else. That they're all focusing on the wrong things. They get upset when they leave their bag on the bus, or their football team loses, or their phone breaks. No one is dying, so don't stress over it. If my car's got a slow puncture or it's leaking coolant. I don't care, I don't! And neither does Mark! I don't care if your shoes are Jimmy Choos or if they're from Primark. Stubbed toes, broken bones, car windshields cracked by stones. Blackheads, dandruff, thread veins, greasy hair. Old coats, scuffed shoes, ripped tights, nothing to wear. Skirts that are tucked into knickers. Saying 'shit' in front of vicars. Posh frocks, toilet's blocked, gone out and the doors unlocked. Makeup that hides your pores. Burst pipes that flood your floors. Gammy knee, burnt tea, traffic jam and need a wee. Chipped tooth, chipped nail. The Turin Shroud, The Holy Grail. The things that get others so riled, mean nothing compared to your child.

I'll accept my nomination for Poet Laureate now.

This whole time, Amy and Friends was going strong, and our conferences were a hit! We were making a difference! Amy won an award, the charity won an award, we were forging ahead. We helped scientists discover the fatal danger of Metronidazole, we were providing help to families, and we were starting to get quite well-known. Our supporters were fantastic, and the number of ways people have found to raise money for us, is astounding. Like the person who climbed Mount Everest in an Amy and Friends t-shirt!

People have been amazing.

And Amy was surrounded by friends. People loved her. I've not talked about this enough in this book because it's not really a medical issue, but my goodness she was friends with some utterly wonderful people.

That doctor who said she'd never have any friends was dead wrong. And what a needless thing to have said! As not only did Amy have masses of friends, she was the one to bring everyone together.

Right. Where were we? Dr Mohammed had been fighting a ten-year battle at this point, trying to get our clinic off the ground. At times it felt like we were getting nowhere. The years were passing, and it didn't seem to be any closer to reality. There were absolutely moments when it felt like there was no way it could happen.

Dr Mohammed recalls:

"In one of the last meetings with NHS England I said, 'You know we keep coming and I will keep fighting, but I need you to tell me, should I just keep coming or is it time to draw a line in the sand?' And they said, 'No, I think we're nearly there.'"

I mean we'd heard that several times, but this time it turned out to be true.

When I got the phone call from Dr Mohammed, I was driving home to North Wales. I answered, hands free, and she just said, 'WE'VE GOT IT! WE'VE GOT IT! WE'VE GOT THE CLINIC!"

It was instant tears for me. I was driving home, but I knew there'd be nobody in, so instead I drove to the tiny little pub in our village. It's a friendly little place, and I had to tell someone. I had to tell everyone! So I ran into the pub, half of them had no idea who I was, and I shouted, 'YOU'RE NOT GOING TO BELIEVE THIS EVERYBODY!"

And that's how my village found out first that our clinic had the go-ahead.

They were brilliant, they cheered and they clapped, and as I celebrated with friends and strangers, I realised, I can die now, and it will all carry on. The kids will get the help they need. That might come across as a bit morbid, but actually, it was the most amazing feeling. It was wonderful.

WE GOT THE CLINIC!

It took so much longer than any of us had anticipated; we had to fight every inch of the way, but it had all been worth it.

This is where Dr Mohammed pulls together the most fantastic team of specialists. She literally cherry-picked the best for us, many of whom had not dealt with Cockayne Syndrome before but were more than up to the challenge. Even if they were retired, if they were the best, we got them. Look at Professor Lehmann and Julia Hopkins. They could be wearing slippers, watching daytime TV, and yelling at youngsters to get off their lawn. But they're not. They're in our clinic twice a month, working their backsides off to give our children the care they deserve.

Dr Mohammed also made sure she found out from the parents just what they wanted to see at the clinic. I'll let her tell you:

"The families of children with Cockayne Syndrome wanted a service where the clinicians that they're seeing are sympathetic. They know the condition is progressive and life-limiting, but they wanted people who will help them look after their children. That led to the development of a model of care where we've made sure all the relevant specialists are present on the day of the clinic."

I cannot tell you how utterly fantastic Dr Mohammed and all of our clinicians are. I'll talk about them later, but it's never not a good time to sing their praises. I wish we had had such amazing doctors throughout Amy's life, and it makes me so very happy that other children, and now adults, have them in our clinic.

Of course, Cockayne Syndrome is a hell of a journey. When the clinic's open day was imminent, Dr Mohammed noticed something wrong in Amy's latest blood test. It was an extremely high level of calcium, indicating an issue with her thyroid. So, she was, in a sense, the first patient the clinic had, as on the opening day, she was taken for a scan.

It wasn't good news.

With Cockayne Syndrome, it's never good news.

It was cancer of the parathyroid.

This meant, realistically, that Amy would only have a year left of life.

Now, I suppose, is the point in this book where we need to talk about death. I'm not a fan of it myself. Zero out of five stars on TripAdvisor, but it happens, and it is something all families with Cockayne Syndrome know they will have to deal with the second their child is diagnosed.

How should you deal with it, as a clinician? Effectively, when you hand out a diagnosis of Cockayne, it's a death sentence, really, isn't it?

Some clinicians clearly really enjoy it. We've had appointments where the clinicians seemed downright gleeful about it. I remember one particular clinician looking like he was getting a buzz out of it when Amy was 16. I thought we were going there for medical help, but instead, he told me we were going to talk about end-of-life plans.

'Not in front of Amy,' I said.

So Amy left the room.

He then proceeded to happily ask me, 'If her stomach explodes, as she's bleeding to death, would you like her to choke to death on her own blood, or would you like us to intervene?'

I mean, Jesus Christ, what a question!

And contrary to one jolly clinician's opinion, end-of-life plans ARE NOT JUST LIKE A BIRTHING PLAN.

Jeez Louise.

Professor Kang answered thoughtfully when asked about talking to patients' parents about how long their child might live:

"One thing that I try not to dwell on too much, especially in early discussions, are topics like life expectancy. The thing that I always tell families is that anything you read about life expectancy is typically a little bit outdated because clinical care is improving constantly. The kids who have Cockayne Syndrome these days, if they go to a children's hospital with a lot of sub-specialists, they get much better care than was available twenty years ago. Whereas the papers that talk about life expectancy were published ten or twenty years ago.

So, that's why I try not to dwell on specific numbers. I tell them that they might find numbers on life expectancy out there, but that information is constantly changing, and new treatments are being developed, so that number may or may not apply to their child.

And I think it's never a good idea to say to a family, 'Your child has X number of years to live, because that, to the family, is like a death sentence. And so then they start counting down the time. So, I really try not to dwell on specific numbers because every child's course is variable. New therapies can be developed, and just routine clinical care improves."

The lovely positive note in all of this, is that thanks to all the hard work done by clinicians, both in the lab and outside of it, our children are living longer, and the quality of their lives is getting better.

Just as one example, look at the way our dietitian, Julia Hopkins, has improved the digestive and bowel horrors that our children suffer from. She's revolutionary in our patients' lives.

I recall towards Amy's end, her problems with constipation were unbearable. Medication wasn't having any impact at all. In fact, it was so agonising, she had started to have seizures on the bathroom floor.

I called the nurse in a panic, not knowing how I could help her, and she laughed at me. She laughed and said, 'You could go for mother and daughter colonics! What a bonding experience that could be!'

Ha ha ha.

Not.

My daughter is dying on the bathroom floor.

Having seizure after seizure.

What a horrific thing for someone to say. Especially someone you are turning to for help.

So you can believe it when I say that the difference Julia Hopkins makes to her patients' lives is worth its weight in gold.

Hang on.

Amy wasn't bothered with gold. When any of her friends asked her what she'd like them to get her for her birthdays, she always answered, 'A photo of you.'

So let's use that as a better measuring system.

The difference Julia Hopkins makes to her patients' lives is worth its weight in photographs of dear friends.

There, much better.

You can see then that things are getting better all the time for people who suffer from Cockayne Syndrome. Their lives are still brutally short, but things are better than they used to be.

Some s*** is still the same, though. Take one of our lovely friends. He was an adult, but Cockayne made him the size of a five-year-old. Despite this, he was treated in an adult hospital ward with adult-sized equipment. And when he needed intubation, the adult-sized tube was so big it caused horrendous injuries to his throat, which subsequently led to the infection that killed him.

Losing him in this way has hit the Amy and Friends community hard. We miss him dearly.

CHAPTER 20: GOODBYE

At the last conference Amy came to, she was struggling. I've told you how upsetting it was to see her so ill. The lovely guys from the Take@That tribute act were devastated when they saw her. But she didn't let it stop her from putting a brave face on it. She was amazing.

Billy Hui's choir, SingMe Merseyside, was there again and they sang Amy's favourite song from their repertoire:

Hallelujah.

At this point, she was so ill she couldn't sing anymore; she could barely even speak. But she began to sing with them. And loudly. She sang and sang, and it was so incredible at this stage of her illness that everyone quietened down to hear her. By the end, everyone was crying. Clapping and crying. Her Nanny and Papa were holding her little hands, overjoyed to hear her voice and see her enjoying every second.

It was one of those beautiful, painful, and poignant moments. None of us shall forget it.

It was December. Her last December, and her voice rang out in that hall. Hundreds of people stopped to listen.

Beautiful.

Since Amy was 22, she had started to go to her best friend's house for Christmas. Ami Knowles had been her friend for a long time; as I said earlier, she'd even lived with us at one point! The first year she spent Christmas with her, it was difficult to get used to. Mark was so upset not to have the whole family around the dinner table. Her brothers and her sister kept asking where she was. I did phone her on Christmas Day, but she was watching a film and didn't want to answer! She was having a brilliant time, and so I thought, let's have a brilliant time too! It's Christmas! And we ended up having a lovely day.

There was just this little voice in the back of my head, however, one that kept saying. 'This is what it's going to feel like when she's gone.'

Her final Christmas, about two days before she went over to her friend's house, she had developed a cough. This was December 2019. It wasn't a particularly bad cough, but she wasn't feeling up to the panto they'd planned to go to. Instead, after insisting that she still went to her friend's house, they decided to stay in and paint their nails.

There wasn't anything strange about her cough that I can put my finger on now. There wasn't any cause for worry.

It just felt different.

Amy's friend was amazing at caring for her. She loved Amy dearly, and she was also pregnant. Amy had always wanted a baby. It broke my heart when she realised at 17 that it could never happen. So, when her best friend became pregnant, she was overjoyed. Ami Knowles' partner was a lovely man, too, who adored our Amy as well.

I had no qualms about Amy being looked after by them, even with a bit of a cough. Ami Knowles had had a sibling pass away from Cockayne Syndrome, so she knew it well.

She knew it well enough that at 8 am on Christmas Eve, she sent me a text that hit like a punch to the gut.

'I think Amy needs to come home and be around her team.'

I walked into Mark's office, where he was working, and said, 'Amy's dying. I'm going to go and get her and bring her home.'

Bless Mark, he told me, full of hope, 'You don't know that.'

But I did.

And I knew Ami Knowles did too. She'd seen it before.

I had to tell my daughter, Laura, on Christmas Eve, I had to tell her, 'Amy's dying. We need to go and get her.'

She held onto the same hope Mark had. And it was devastating to see. The drive was long, on the motorway, with Ami Knowles driving towards us to meet us halfway.

When we reached the meeting point, Amy was lying on the backseat, supported by her friend's partner. She was so sick that when I lifted her out of the car, she was like a rag doll. I tried to put her hand on her best friend's pregnant belly, a sort of goodbye to the child she would never meet, but her hand kept dropping, and I couldn't do it.

Poor Ami Knowles and poor Laura were hysterical. I laid Amy down on the backseat with her sister and I drove like mad, crying, both of us, all the way home.

Mark was shocked to see her. She looked so diminished that no hope could be held out for her. We laid her in her bed, and I called the doctor, who came out to see her. He walked into her room, where her little brother Ben was standing, watching over his sister, took one look at her and said, 'Why is she here? She should be in the hospice. She's end of life.'

That's exactly what he said. In front of Ben. In front of Amy herself.

End of life.

I knew it, but hearing those words is a different thing.

Amy had said that when she went to heaven, she wanted to go in her own bed, listening to music. So taking her into hospice wasn't something I jumped at. Plus, it was Christmas Eve. The doctor said it'd be hard to get her in anywhere. So, he instead gave her an injection, which he said was to calm her down.

But she was calm.

She was so very calm.

Then the doctor laughed and said he'd send somebody around tomorrow to administer the rest of the medication.

I gave Amy her usual 1 ml of morphine that night. She had been taking it for six months. I had been told I could give her as much as 5 ml in an emergency, but it was a terrifying amount that I wasn't ready to try.

That night, I slept next to her in her bed. Ben came in too, and we held each other and cried.

The next morning was Christmas Day. Laura came into her room with matching elf dresses for her and Amy, and she wanted to change Amy into hers. We left her to it but heard her shouting down the stairs that she'd managed to get Amy to drink something! Apple juice! She'd syringed 5 ml of apple juice into Amy's mouth, and she'd swallowed it.

Laura was just 16 years old. 16 years old and excited that she'd managed to get her dying sister to swallow 5 ml of apple juice. It's not fair, is it? It's not fair that a 16-year-old should go through this. This whole thing. It wasn't fair to any of us but watching my baby girl take care of her big sister as she lay dying, it was fucking heartbreaking.

We went through the motions that day, but Amy couldn't even recognise her Christmas presents. We'd bought her this little red and black leopard print fur coat that she'd wanted, and cherry red matching Doc Martins. She didn't respond. She wasn't, she wasn't really there.

I ended up going into the kitchen to cook the dinner and cry. Amy lay on the sofa with her brothers and sister.

The last words that came out of Amy's mouth were because Laura had asked her what she was going to have on her Christmas dinner.

Her answer?

Five pigs in blankets.

That's my girl.

At dinner time obviously she couldn't eat them, but she had a little bit of mashed-up carrot and gravy, and one teaspoon of the lemon posset I'd made specifically because it would be soft enough for her to swallow.

She was trying.

She was trying for us.

Then her breathing worsened. She started to get agitated. The doctor had said someone would come around with medication. But nobody did. Nobody came.

In the end, she was struggling so much I realised I'd have to give her the full 5 ml of morphine. I didn't know, though, I didn't know if it'd kill her. I'd never given her so much, so I told the family to witness it because I didn't want to go to prison for killing her.

I gave her the 5 ml, but she was out of it. Sleeping so deeply, I had to keep touching her to see if she was still breathing, I was terrified I'd killed her with the morphine.

I finally rang the hospice and I told them, 'I can't do this. If the doctor isn't going to come with the medication, if nobody comes today with it, I can't do this at home.'

They told me there'd be a bed free for her tomorrow. A family room. It was a lovely hospice. We'd been going every week, for the raffle or to get her nails done. One time they'd shown us around and had taken us from the day care into the actual hospice, and Amy had pointed to that very room and said, 'I'm going to stay in that room one day.'

That night, everyone slept in Amy's room. All of us, me, Mark, Jonny, Ben, and Laura.

That's not fair to any of them, is it, that they had to go through this.

The next morning we drove her as fast as we could to the hospice. I held her in the back seat with her dear friend Aleisha, who had come running when we called her. Mark lifted her from the car and carried her in his arms into the hospice with such love and care.

I remember how he carried her into that pub when she was so young, declaring to everyone, 'This is my Amy. Isn't she wonderful?'

This time, he was carrying her to her final journey.

It was more than I could bear then, and it is more than I can bear now.

I struggled knowing she wanted to die at home, but we didn't have the medication. They didn't bring it when they said they would. It wasn't possible to take her pain away at home. At the hospice they had the medication she needed, and they gave it to her the moment she looked like she was hurting. They looked after her so well. We couldn't have done that at home. Not without the medication.

They all knew us in the day care in that hospice, so many of the staff were popping in to see her and crying too when they saw how different she looked to even two weeks ago. They put photos of her up in the room so the hospice staff could see who she was, who she used to be until this moment.

She was Amy. She was Amy, who used to carry herself with such strength, and dignity, and utterly glorious bald-faced cheek.

She wasn't this girl lying in this bed. This wasn't the sum of who she was. She was so much more. She was everything to us.

We decorated her hospice room just like her bedroom at home. The hospice staff were wonderful about it.

We all stayed with her in that room, by her side. She held on for a week. It was an horrific time, but we did our best. We played games she loved to play, and pretended she was joining in.

We didn't know if we should feed her or not. We were thinking perhaps she needed the strength to get through this, to die. It sounds silly, I suppose, but we'd never been through this before. We didn't know what to do. In the end, we put a little formula down her feeding tube, but it came back up, out of her mouth, and it seemed to cause her so much pain that we stopped.

We didn't know if it was the formula or if it was a one off. So later we tried again, with the tiniest bit of her favourite Milky Bar pudding. It happened again.

Her stomach had failed.

Laura had a little sponge to wet Amy's mouth. She dipped it into Dr Pepper and Coke, Amy's favourites, which she wasn't allowed too often, and she dabbed her mouth with that instead of water.

By this point it was impossible to get Amy comfortable. She had bed sores and we tried our best to move her to stop them, but it didn't work. They were awful. The final time we moved her, her hip bone came through the skin. It came right through the skin of my precious girl, and I couldn't, I couldn't handle it anymore. I called the nurse and told her, 'We can't see any more of this. We're done. You need to take over from us now.'

As she lay there dying, it was such a beautiful day outside. It was New Year's Day. The sun was shining in through the window and onto her face. She had always loved the sun on her face, and I whispered to her, 'The sun is on your face, Amy. You love that.'

Outside the window of her ground floor room, two rabbits, two squirrels, and white doves were in the gardens. They were so close to her window, it was like something out of Snow White. It was heart-wrenching and beautiful and awful and painful, and it will never leave me. Not one second of it. I carry it with me, and it will stay with me forever. Just like Amy's bathrobe that still hangs on the back of the bathroom door.

I had sent the boys off home to grab a quick shower, and while they were gone, while the rest of us held onto her, Mark, my mum, Laura, Ami Knowles, Aleisha, and me, she passed away. Jonny and Ben were devastated by that, but I didn't know, I didn't know that would be the moment she would die. She had been on the brink for a week, but I know that upset them deeply.

She was gone.

She was gone.

Amy was gone.

We sat with her. The hospice couldn't get hold of a second doctor on New Year's Day to sign off on the paperwork, so Mark and I slept alongside her that night.

We had new pyjamas for her to wear. The top had a teddy bear on it, and the bottoms were leopard print. Laura, Ami Knowles, and Aleisha ran home to fetch matching knickers. Matching leopard print knickers.

Our Amy loved wearing matching knickers.

We gave it all to the funeral director to dress her in, who was a kind friend of ours.

The second doctor turned up that day. Over 24 hours after she had passed. They declared her dead for a charge of £84. A nurse described this to us as "Ashes for Cashes". It didn't seem right or appropriate or in any way sensitive, but it's what happened.

And they took Amy away.

We drove home, but we didn't want to go back into the house. It was hard. It was so damn hard.

She was wonderful.

She was Amy.

I loved her. Her family loved her. Everyone loved her.

When she sang, hundreds of people hushed just to hear her.

Her impact on the world has been huge, and her legacy helps thousands of people around the globe. And I keep it together, I push on and help other families go through what we went through, but the pain of losing her will never leave me.

At her funeral, we sang her favourite, Hallelujah. I will forever associate that song with her. Every time I hear it, I hear her again.

I still hear you, Amy.

Since Amy has passed away, I have been there for countless families as their child lies dying. I hold their hands. I try to give them strength in the way Amy showed me how. When a single father called me to tell me his daughter was choking to death, I stayed on the phone with him, I was there for him. And with every single child that dies, I'm thrown back into the fear, the panic, the dread, and the pain that I experienced when I lost Amy. And I will never stop. I will never stop rushing to the side of families whose children are dying.

I will make them strong.

Just as Amy made me strong.

CHAPTER 21: THE CLINIC

Every member of the family handled their grief differently, and I don't think any of us coped well. Jonny went back to his university flat. Ben was living with his girlfriend at the time. Laura stayed home, and Aleisha stayed with her. Mark locked himself away in his office. I was desperate to talk about it all, but their grief couldn't bear to hear it.

It wasn't a happy house at all, which is absolutely not what Amy would have wanted, but we couldn't help it.

The hospice offered us half an hour of counselling every Wednesday for six weeks. That's not even seven minutes for every year of Amy's life. I don't know. It's not enough, is it? It's like pissing on a forest fire.

Grief is a massive part of Cockayne Syndrome, and our clinic takes it seriously. There's grief after your child's initial diagnosis, grief every time their condition deteriorates, grief when you try to come to terms with how short their life will be, and grief when they pass away and leave us behind.

We have some amazing psychologists and counsellors. Plus, we work with a group called Love, Jasmine. Love, Jasmine was set up by the parents of a little girl who passed away when she was just six years old. She didn't have an underlying condition. She asphyxiated on a grape. It devastated them, and they ended up setting up a charity for bereaved parents and siblings. When we started working with them, I asked if they could also train in anticipatory grief, and so they did. They're phenomenal, and every counsellor in that group has lost a child. So, they know, don't they, how it feels. The hospice counsellor, who offered us half an hour on Wednesdays, and who seemed to disappear any time any of us even thought about talking to her, had never lost a child. The difference is huge.

It's hard all around, but Love, Jasmine really helps. They are so kind. They're excellent.

We also have Rewired For Men, a mental health group for dads who struggle with the grieving process. Often, men find it hard to be vulnerable. Society says they have to be the strong ones, and many fathers internalise this, feeling like they're letting everyone down if they can't cope, or they find it difficult to keep working throughout it all. Their dads' group creates a safe space for fathers to speak freely and actually, by allowing themselves to be vulnerable, by not turning to destructive behaviour, or blaming others, they become stronger than they ever were. They're a kind bunch. I recommend them.

As for me, in the end, the only counselling I got was speaking to someone on the internet, although they did say something that hit home. I had just told them that I had known that Amy wasn't going to live long. I said it almost as if it meant perhaps, I shouldn't have been hit by it so hard.

They said, 'If I told you I was going to punch you in the face, it won't hurt any less when I do it.'

Up until that point, I'd felt almost guilty about grieving so hard. After all, other children in Amy and Friends pass away so very much younger. Sometimes as young as four-years-old. And I had known, hadn't I, since she was two, that she would live a short life. However, speaking to that kind person online helped me ditch that baggage and just grieve.

Three months later, the UK went into lockdown. COVID-19 shut everything down. Our families at Amy and Friends were hit hard. Parents were furloughed, many of them struggled to buy food and heat the house. I threw myself into helping them, and in a way, that helped me get through Amy's death. Perhaps it still does.

We had a lot of work to keep our families going. Lockdown was difficult for everyone, especially people with kids. However, for people with children who had disabilities, it was really bloody hard. Amy and Friends sent money and food to struggling families. We sent out 26,000 activity packs to keep the kids entertained. We held online barmy bingo sessions with DJ Keith and family parties. I sent ingredients for things like shortbread to their houses and then met them all online to show them how to make scrumptious treats.

In short, I went into overdrive. And we got through that bloody awful year that was 2020.

When lockdown ended, our clinic opened up again, and it's been amazing. It's changed everything for our families! We pay for five families to travel to London twice a month. We organise their transport, we contact the trains so they have help, or we send volunteers to help them travel. We also make sure the kids have fun goody bags to play with while travelling. Then we pay for their taxi from the train station to the hotel.

We put them up in the Premier Inn, by Westminster Bridge. It's a three-minute walk to the clinic from there, and the staff are wonderful. They always welcome us, to the point where they're practically part of the family. When I showed up there for the first time without Amy, the kind man who works there asked me, 'Where the lovely little girl was?' When I told him she'd passed away, he held my hands and cried.

You don't get that kind of service at the Ritz, do you?

We all then gather together for dinner. An anticipatory grief counsellor comes along to talk to the parents while we help feed the kids and play. The kids especially love that because so many of them have never met another child like them. They bond so quickly because of it.

Sometimes the kids are too excited to go to bed that night, but the real fun starts the next day at the clinic.

I help feed the kids breakfast. Many of the children are tube-fed, and those who can eat only eat a very small amount and take a long time over it. So we help there and let the parents eat in peace. Our carers all step in here and they're brilliant with the children.

One of our carers, Meg, has lots of experience working with children with special needs. She is incredible with them. She can calm down an agitated child in seconds. A sweet girl who came to clinic was blind, and I watched Meg put this little girl's hand on her wrist, where she wore a bracelet, and tell her, 'I'm Meg. Feel my bracelet. I'm Meg with the bracelet.' The next time she came over to her, she put the girl's hand on her wrist, and the lovely little girl exclaimed, 'Meg! With the bracelet!'

It was such a simple thing. It was such a small thing. Yet at the same time, it was huge.

Choosing Meg to be one of our carers was an easy job. She impressed us by raising £60,000 in six weeks by applying for grants. She has since impressed us by keeping everything running smoothly during conferences, and by her sick moves on the dance floor. She's bloody hilarious, full of energy, and has a tendency to lose her bumbag whilst still wearing it.

So, Meg, our other brilliant carers, and I help the kids eat breakfast, and there's always so much laughter, it's like an amazing birthday party.

Then we all head over to the clinic, and it's phlebotomy first. You know by now the horror phlebotomy is for children with Cockayne Syndrome, and they do get nervous at our clinic. However, at the same time, they're so excited to go upstairs where we have a party, that they're eager to get in and out of phlebotomy.

We have a big table up there where we have all the arts and crafts you could imagine, plus toys. Meg always buys new sensory toys and half the time it's the doctors playing with them. That's when they're not doing Superman. It was Meg, by the way, who lifted Professor Alan Lehmann, the distinguished geneticist, into the air.

I think I shall show that video at our next conference. The clinicians will love it.

It goes without saying that throughout the time we are all at clinic, cups of tea abound.

With biscuits.

The nurses are brilliant, they measure the kids and take their blood pressure, and they don't mind having it done because we're with them and they're having fun. They're in and out of rooms seeing specialists all morning. We have a timetable, but we don't have to stick to it. If one of our specialists needs more time with a patient, they can go ahead and take as much time as they'd like. If families are nervous and want me or one of our carers to go into any of the appointments with them, we do.

We also take photographs to capture the difference in the children over time. We make sure to take pictures of their faces, hands, and feet.

Dr Mohammed talks about what our clinic entails:

"Our patients see up to ten specialists in one day. It means that we can organise an efficient flow whereby all the children are seen by all the relevant specialists. We'll be organising up to fifty appointments just in the morning alone, so it involves a lot of planning. We make sure, though, that it meets the needs of the children.'

Then, it's lunch!

We give the families lunch vouchers for different restaurants and cafes nearby. They can go and eat, or we can get them food to go. If the morning appointments have run on, we'll nip to M&S and get a whole buffet for them to eat at the clinic.

After lunch, there aren't many appointments left

And then all the clinicians come together.

This is where the magic happens. They all come together and discuss each patient and the multidisciplinary care they need. They'll formulate a plan going forward and contact each child's local doctors to let them know how to proceed.

Every child's case is looked at in detail.

Anything that can be done, is done.

It's wonderful.

The families then go home. It's usually a late night for them, so I wait until Monday, and then I phone them to see how they're all doing. We get feedback too, and so far, it's stellar, which helps us to get our grants.

Our clinic even takes care of the children when they're not in London. Parents can phone us if they need help or advice. If a child needs emergency surgery and their local hospital can't fit them in, we bring them over to London to get it done there.

Plus, we investigate the disorder as a whole. Our brilliant nurses collate all of the information which makes it possible to spot patterns, such as the increased number of deaths in the winter. It seemed with all the coughs and colds, our children were particularly susceptible to catching them and developing an infection. So, we've introduced prophylactic antibiotics, just for the colder months and its impact has been huge.

The more patients we see, the more we learn. We are always looking for patterns that can help us predict our children's needs. Plus, we can implement change fast.

Sometimes our lovely patients are too ill to come to clinic. That's when one of our nurses will travel to their house, and then all the appointments will be conducted with the clinic online. However, every patient also starts off their journey with us with a home visit. Phillipa Sellar talked to me about it for this book:

"Part of the service proposal was for home visits by nurses to create a holistic nursing assessment that can then be transcribed into a bespoke care plan. So, a home visit, when it's a new patient, consists of a three-hour visit, where we, with the child/young persons at the centre of a holistic assessment, with their family, identify an individual's care needs."

So yes, we know about their genetic condition, and we know about a diagnosis, but what are the specific needs of the individual? From that home visit, we create a bespoke set of patient-held documents, including a healthcare passport. The second part of it is an acute care plan, tailored to the diagnosis, giving medical support. This also contains guidance around calorie intake and fluid overload because it's very difficult for clinicians who have been trained in a certain way to undo that thinking. For example, most drugs, once you get over the age of ten or eleven, are age-specific. Not weight-specific. So this care plan would have a lot around the correct fluid intake and drug intake for this specific child."

But when it comes to contact, we go even further than that. Here's Dr Mohammed to tell you about it:

"The appointment in the hospital is not the only contact that the families have. We are very approachable, we are accessible. So if there is a query that we can help with, they can contact the nursing team or me and we will try and facilitate whatever the medical issue is. Then we follow up after the appointment, because as you can imagine, it can be quite overwhelming, particularly for parents who are coming for the first time, as they may be seeing children who are perhaps slightly older than their own child, which can be quite difficult for some families, understandably.

But we do follow that up with a phone call or a video call to make sure any questions they might have can be resolved. And then, in between the hospital, the nursing team visits the child at home."

If you want to know more about this, please do contact us and sign up to our newsletter:

https://amyandfriends.org/contact/

https://amyandfriends.org/amy-and-friends-newsletter/

There, do you see?

We listen.

We diagnose.

And by God do we care.

We care about every single one of them—the children with Cockayne Syndrome, their siblings, and their parents. We care about them all.

Right from the moment we set up the Amy and Friends charity, we put caring right into the heart of it. It determines everything we do. And we have had an epic journey so far. I was awarded the British Empire Medal! I got a new dress for it and everything. Our clinic keeps going from strength to strength, and our conferences grow in size every year. We have some of the best minds in the world working for us. And you've seen in this book the trajectory on which we're heading. Things are getting better all the time for our children. More kids are getting diagnosed younger. There's more understanding of how to manage their symptoms. They're living longer. We're helping the NHS. We're helping the families. And we make it fun.

In the grand scheme of things, when faced with the enormous impact Cockayne Syndrome has on the body, the sheer number of symptoms it causes, and the grief it leaves behind, having fun might seem like a very small thing.

But the small things.

The small things are the most important things of all.

Hallelujah.

EPILOGUE

To those of you that I leave behind, I know you'll cry for me. I want you to cry for a little bit, and then I want you to stop and live your lives. Make sure you live them well.

Do as I once could: dance, light up the room, sing as loud as you can, who cares if you're not in tune! Take time for your friends, have a cuppa with them, tea was my favourite, two sugars (Mum, I know you only put half a teaspoon in, but I made everyone else put two!) Take joy from the smallest of things, and most of all love with all of your heart.

Amy

ABOUT THE AUTHOR

Jayne Hughes BEM

Jayne Hughes was born in North Wales and lived for many years on the Wirral before returning to her birthplace. She was expecting a normal life, like everyone else; she worked for an insurance company, for crying out loud! However, her life decided it was going to go off-piste and hurtle towards the unknown when her daughter, Amy, was born with atypical Cockayne Syndrome/XRCC4. It took 14 long years before Amy was finally diagnosed, and by that time, Jayne wasn't just off-piste, she was facing an avalanche.

That avalanche was a lack of support from professionals, limited research and interest in Cockayne Syndrome, and diagnostic difficulties.

Her response?

She set up Amy and Friends, a UK-based charity (registered charity no. 1119746) that supports children and families affected by Cockayne Syndrome and other DNA repair disorders. First, she organised annual conferences for families and interested scientists. Then, with help from a couple of distinguished geneticists, she helped establish Rare Disease Clinics in the UK and the Netherlands (in partnership with NHS England/Guy's and St Thomas' NHS Foundation Trust).

Hundreds of families have been helped.

Scientific research has progressed at a phenomenal rate.

Whether you're a patient, a family member, a scientist, or a local GP, Amy and Friends makes sure you're not traversing through the world of DNA repair disorders alone. The charity offers practical, medical, and psychological help. Plus, it offers friendship.

Jayne's wonderful husband, Mark, and brilliant children, Amy, Jonny, Ben, and Laura, have all played a large part in her success. They are behind every step forward the charity makes.

Jayne has won many awards for the difference she's made to people affected by Cockayne Syndrome.

The avalanche is still coming, but Jayne refuses to get snowed under. She'll dig her way out with her British Empire Medal if she has to.

CONNECT WITH US

Website
https://amyandfriends.org/

Contact us
https://amyandfriends.org/contact/

Join our newsletter
https://amyandfriends.org/amy-and-friends-newsletter/

Facebook
https://www.facebook.com/amyandfriendsCockayneSyndromeandTTD

Instagram
https://www.instagram.com/amyandfriends_cs_ttd/

Tik Tok
https://www.tiktok.com/@amyandfriendstiktok

X

https://x.com/AmyandFriends
Linked IN
https://www.linkedin.com/company/amyandfriends/posts/?feedView=all
https://www.linkedin.com/in/jayne-hughes-4a713325b/
You Tube
https://www.youtube.com/@AmyandFriendsWorldwide

www.ingramcontent.com/pod-product-compliance
Lightning Source LLC
Chambersburg PA
CBHW051548020426
42333CB00016B/2152